WHAT YOU MUST KNOW ABOUT
KIDNEY DISEASE

A PRACTICAL GUIDE TO USING CONVENTIONAL AND COMPLEMENTARY TREATMENTS

RICH SNYDER, DO

D0963076

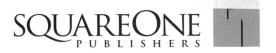

SQUAREONE
PUBLISHERS

The information and advice contained in this book are based upon the research and the personal and professional experiences of the author. They are not intended as a substitute for consulting with a health care professional. The publisher and author are not responsible for any adverse effects or consequences resulting from the use of any of the suggestions, preparations, or procedures discussed in this book. All matters pertaining to your physical health should be supervised by a health care professional. It is a sign of wisdom, not cowardice, to seek a second or third opinion.

COVER DESIGNER: Jeannie Tudor
EDITOR: Anna Comstock
TYPESETTER: Gary A. Rosenberg

Square One Publishers
115 Herricks Road • Garden City Park, NY 11040
(516) 535-2010 • (877) 900-BOOK
www.squareonepublishers.com

**25% of all proceeds received for this book
will be donated to the American Kidney Fund.**

Library of Congress Cataloging-in-Publication Data
Snyder, Rich.
  What you must know about kidney disease : a practical guide to using conventional and complementary treatments / Rich Snyder.
     p. cm.
  Includes bibliographical references.
  ISBN 978-0-7570-0326-4
  1. Kidneys—Diseases—Popular works. 2. Kidneys—Diseases—Treatment--Popular
works. 3. Kidneys—Diseases—Alternative treatment—Popular works. I. Title.
  RC902.S62 2010
  616.6'1—dc22
                    2010025610

Printed in Canada

10   9   8   7   6   5   4   3   2   1

Contents

Acknowledgments, vi

Introduction, 1

PART ONE   **An Introduction to Kidney Disease**

1. An Overview of Kidney Function and
   How It Is Evaluated, 5

2. Setting the Stage of Kidney Disease—
   Where Do You Stand? 19

3. Interacting with Healthcare Professionals, 27

PART TWO   **Inflammation, Causes of Kidney Disease,
             and Standard Treatments**

4. The Inflammatory Response, Oxidative Stress,
   and the Kidneys, 37

5. Common Causes of Kidney Disease, 45

6. Other Conditions That Can Affect the Kidneys, 65

7. Medications, Imaging Studies, and Interventions, 75

8. Complications of Chronic Kidney Disease and
   Standard Treatment Approaches, 85

PART THREE   **Complementary Treatment Approaches
and Lifestyle Changes**

9. Lifestyle Changes Everyone Can Make,   93

10. The Importance of Eating Right,   105

11. Vitamins, Minerals, and Other Nutritional
Supplements,   125

12. Herbs and Complementary Therapies,   135

13. Spiritual and Emotional Components of Healing,   149

Conclusion,   157

Glossary,   158

Resources,   161

References,   167

Index, 181

To my mother, Nancy Snyder,
I dedicate this book.
Without her help and support,
I would not have been able to do this.

I also dedicate this book
to anyone with kidney disease.
You are the real heroes.

Acknowledgments

There are many people out there who have been beacons of light and have helped me along the way. I am proud to call them mentors, but more importantly, to call them friends and family.

For helping give me my start in Nephrology, I personally thank from the bottom of my heart Dr. Raph Cohen. You helped this "big lug" in more ways than one.

For having a great bunch of people to work with at LVNA, I say thank you all for being the great people that you are.

To Patty Paul, one of the best nurses I have ever had the privilege of working with and calling my friend, you are missed but never, ever forgotten. You live on in our hearts.

To Rudy Shur and everyone at Square One, thank you for giving me the opportunity to write this book. To Anna, thank you for being a terrific editor.

To all of the wonderful nurses and patients that I have had the privilege of knowing, thank you for allowing me into your lives. I am a much better man for it.

In an effort to avoid awkward phrasing within sentences, it is our publishing style to alternate the use of generic male and female pronouns according to chapter. This means that when referring to a "third-person" patient or caregiver, odd-numbered chapters will use female pronouns, while even-numbered chapters will use male.

$\mathcal{I}$ntroduction

The fear, anxiety, and disbelief induced by hearing that you have kidney disease can be overwhelming. After the initial shock, however, you begin searching for vital information: What is kidney disease? What are its silent signs and symptoms? And how can it best be treated?

Deciding on the best options for treatment includes understanding both standard medical therapy and alternative treatments. Armed with that information, better treatment choices for yourself or your loved one can be made.

What You Must Know About Kidney Disease will empower you by providing you with necessary information so that you, with your doctor, can make the best treatment decisions possible. As you read this book, you will learn many things you can do to positively impact your kidney health and overall well-being—from dietary changes to lifestyle modification. Gaining insight into your kidney health will enable you to ask your doctor relevant questions pertaining to your treatment plan, in order to learn what works best for you.

This book is structured to give you a holistic view of the treatment of kidney disease. In addition to standard medical therapy, you will read about complementary approaches to give you a truly informed perspective. Part One of this book covers the basics: where the kidneys are, what they do, and the important role they play in maintaining your overall health. In addition to being your body's filters, they are also important in the preservation of your blood, bone, and heart health. You'll discover what is meant by kidney disease, as well as the various stages doctors use to define it. You'll read about ways to maximize an office visit with your kidney doctor and other health care providers. And finally, your healthcare team and your role as captain of that team will be explored in detail.

In Part Two, you'll discover that kidney disease is a state of inflammation that can affect other organs of the body, specifically the heart. In addition, you'll also learn about management and treatment of other common diseases, such as hypertension and diabetes, that affect kidney function. Part Two also reviews other causes of kidney disease including obesity, atherosclerosis, and polycystic kidney disease, as well as provides a detailed discussion of an important group of conditions that are called the high-level inflammatory syndromes. You'll learn about the potential dangers of commonly ordered imaging tests, such as MRI and CAT scans, and invasive procedures, such as the cardiac catheterization.

In Part Three, we'll examine lifestyle modifications that everyone, regardless of their stage of kidney disease, can make to improve their kidney function and their lives. You will understand the role that nutrition plays and its relationship to kidney health, as well as the role of vitamin and herbal supplementation. Kidney cleansing will be discussed, as well as the many benefits of complementary therapies, including osteopathic manipulation (osteopathy), homeopathy, and acupuncture. Lastly, the all-important emotional and spiritual component of healing will be examined. The role of a strong belief system and family support cannot be emphasized enough in the healing process.

Your kidney health is important and you need to be a major participant in your own healthcare. Members of your healthcare team should include your kidney doctor, your primary care doctor, and other healthcare providers to achieve the best outcome. The information contained in this book will allay your fears and arm you with the knowledge you need, so let's begin!

PART ONE

---

*A*n Introduction to Kidney Disease

The kidneys are our bodies' unsung heroes and are vital to helping us maintain our health and vitality. They do so many important things and their actions affect our bodies' many systems. Part One of this book is geared toward introducing you to the kidneys and all of the wonderful things that they do. In the first chapter, you will not only begin to understand the functions of the kidneys, but you will also learn what kidney disease is and how our bodies are affected by it. You will gain an insight into the various types of blood work and other testing that doctors often use to diagnose kidney disease. And you will begin to understand that kidney disease is indeed a matter of epidemic proportions, as it affects millions of people.

Chapter 2 serves to answer the question: I know I have kidney disease, but how severe is it? This chapter will take you through the various stages doctors use to define kidney disease and their progression. Early intervention and treatment by a kidney doctor is the key to preventing a worsening to the next stage. An in-depth look at protein in the urine and its role in affecting kidney function is presented, and you will also read about the importance of preparing for dialysis and undergoing a kidney transplant evaluation at the very advanced stages of kidney disease.

In Chapter 3, the final chapter in Part One, you will learn about the members of your care healthcare team, including your kidney doctor, and the important and supportive roles they play in your care. Healthcare in kidney disease is a team effort, but you as the patient are the most important member of that team. As such, you will gain much-needed insight about how to best maximize a visit with your kidney doctor and other health care professionals.

1

$\mathcal{A}$n Overview of Kidney Function and How It Is Evaluated

T he nature of the human body is one of balance. Similar to the musical instruments of a beautiful symphony, the mind and all of the body's systems passionately maintain this harmony. The lungs provide us with life-sustaining oxygen, the heart continually pumps nutrient-rich blood throughout the body, and the kidneys are the body's filters, purifiers, and unsung heroes. This book is dedicated to the kidneys—the two, bean-shaped organs that are vital in maintaining the body's perfect state of physical and mental balance. In this chapter, you will receive several answers to frequently asked questions about kidney disease.

WHERE ARE THE KIDNEYS LOCATED?

The kidneys are located behind the belly, one on either side of the spinal column. They are found underneath the ribs right where your mid-back (thoracic spine) meets your lower back (lumbar spine). The right kidney sits a little lower than the left. In an average-sized person, the kidneys are approximately four inches in length, but their size can vary depending on a person's body size, and degree and duration of kidney disease.

Each kidney is connected to a small, tube-like structure called a *ureter (your-i-ter)* that serves as a bridge between the kidney and bladder. Urine is formed in the kidneys, and then it flows through the ureters into the bladder, which is the temporary holding tank. When the bladder is full, the urine exits the body through another tube-like structure called the *urethra (your-wreath-ra)*. Together, the kidneys, ureters, bladder, and urethra make up the body's urinary tract, as shown in Figure 1.1.

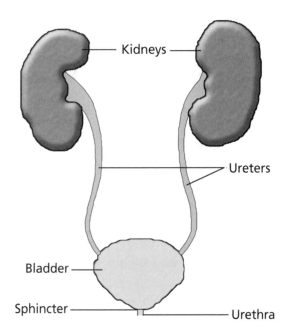

Figure 1.1. Front view of the urinary tract.

WHAT DO THE KIDNEYS DO?

As the body's filters, the kidneys clean and purify the blood by eliminating toxins as waste. Think of a pool pump filter. The pool water flows into the pump and through the filter, where the waste products are removed. The filtered water is then pumped back into the pool. In the body, blood flows into the kidneys where the toxins are removed. Unlike the pool analogy, however, after the blood is filtered, the by-product—urine—is excreted.

The kidneys are composed of millions of small blood filters, called *glomeruli (glo-mare-ewl-eye)*, working together to clean your blood twenty-four hours a day, seven days a week. When we discuss kidney function, the actual focus is on how well these small filters are collectively doing their job. In other words, in evaluating kidney function, your doctor is looking for the answer to one question: *How well are the kidneys functioning as filters?*

Additionally, the kidneys have a kind of "sixth sense," in that as they filter the blood, they instinctively know when the body is out of balance. When it is, the kidneys correct it. For example, if we eat too much sodium in our diet, normally functioning kidneys will remove the excess sodium the body doesn't need; thereby keeping the body in balance. In much the same way, the kidneys are programmed to keep blood levels of the minerals potassium, calcium, and magnesium within a normal range. These basic, life-sustaining ingredients are called *electrolytes (elek-tro-lites)*. Regulation of their levels is important to maintaining total body balance.

The Kidneys and Acid-Base Balance

In addition to those previously listed, another important electrolyte is *bicarbonate (bye-carb-o-net)*, which is your body's equivalent of baking soda—a very strong base. Going back to the pool analogy, every pool owner learns how to maintain the proper acid/base—or pH—levels of the pool water. In a similar way, the kidneys' role is to maintain the body's acid/base balance.

Changes in this balance, such as too much acid and a low amount of bicarbonate, can influence how well the other organs of the body function. Malfunctioning kidneys can cause bicarbonate levels to fall. When this happens, the acid level in the blood can build up, and over a period of time, the high acid levels can be toxic to the body.

The Kidneys and Blood Pressure

The kidneys also help in regulating blood pressure. In addition to eliminating excess sodium from the body, which helps in maintaining a normal blood pressure, they are responsible for the production of certain blood pressure hormones called *renin (wren-in)* and *angiotensin (angie-o-tense-in)*. The kidneys make these two hormones when the blood pressure is low. Moreover, the *adrenal (a-dree-null)* gland, which sits on top of the kidneys, makes a third hormone called *aldosterone (al-dost-tair-own)*. The job of all three of these hormones is to raise the blood pressure.

Unfortunately, these hormones—referred to as the renin-angiotensin-aldosterone (RAA) system—can also adversely affect the kidneys. As you'll read in Chapter 4, these hormones can elicit inflammatory changes in the kidneys of those with kidney disease, as well as contribute to the worsening of kidney function for people with high blood pressure, diabetes, and the many other conditions that cause kidney disease.

The Kidneys as Regulators of Blood and Bone Health

The kidneys are major players in maintaining both blood and bone health, as well. To keep the blood healthy, they produce a hormone called *erythropoietin (erith-ro-po-eaten)*, which is a kind of "blood stimulator." This hormone fuels the production of blood cells in the body and is important for keeping the blood count normal. To keep the bones healthy, the kidneys transform and "activate" vitamin D obtained from both diet and sun exposure. Vitamin D is responsible for preserving bone, heart, and total body health. Unfortunately, many of us in this country are deficient in this important vitamin. Proper supplementation of this essential vitamin is crucial, and will be discussed further in Chapter 11.

WHAT IS KIDNEY DISEASE?

Kidney disease refers to any condition that, over time, affects the kidneys' ability to do their job as filters. There are many conditions that can affect kidney function, but a discussion of all of them is beyond the scope of this book. Instead, we will focus on the most common causes, which, in this country, are hypertension (high blood pressure) and diabetes. Obesity, which has become an epidemic in itself, is also a cause. Some conditions that affect kidney function, like diabetes, are obtained during one's lifetime, whereas others, like polycystic kidney disease, can be inherited from family members. Common causes of kidney disease are discussed in more detail in Part Two. For now, the focus is on three important questions that patients commonly ask about it.

Timing and Duration of Kidney Disease

The first question commonly asked by patients about kidney disease is, *how long have I had it?* The doctor's response is based on the results of blood tests. Upon reviewing the patient's blood work, the doctor will classify the duration of the patient's kidney disease as either acute or chronic. Acute kidney disease refers to any condition that worsens kidney function quickly, over a period of several hours or days. Chronic kidney disease (CKD), on the other hand, refers to a change in kidney function that occurs over weeks or months, and doesn't return to normal. There are many conditions that affect the kidney acutely at first, before resulting in a long-term or chronic problem. Therefore, for the purposes of this book, the term "kidney disease" will be referring to CKD, unless otherwise specified.

Severity of Kidney Disease

Another common question is, *how bad are my kidneys?* This is such a loaded, complex question that the entire next chapter is devoted to answering it.

Chronic Kidney Disease (CKD)— A Matter of Epidemic Proportions

Finally, a third question patients often ask is, *do other people have problems with their kidneys?* The answer is yes—millions of people do. More than twenty-six million people in this country have been diagnosed with CKD, and this staggering number continues to grow.

This statistic may even be an underestimation, as it cannot take into account the thousands, or even millions more people that still remain undiagnosed. And what's more, common causes of kidney disease like diabetes, hypertension, and obesity, which were once thought to be conditions of "older people," are now affecting younger generations, including many teenagers. Thus, the upward trend of CKD diagnoses is likely to continue.

HOW DO I KNOW IF I HAVE KIDNEY DISEASE?

Often, the first sign of a kidney problem will be an abnormality in your blood work, which will be discussed in more detail a little later in this chapter. If you see your doctor on a regular basis, chances are you have had routine blood work done. If that is the case, keep getting it done at least once a year. If you have never had blood work done, now is the time to start.

Many of my patients, after hearing about their abnormal blood test results, will ask, "I feel okay and I urinate fine, so how can there be a problem with my kidneys?" The fact is that many people with both mild and advanced kidney disease may not experience any symptoms at all.

This is one of the major concerns kidney doctors face. *Some people can feel perfectly normal, yet have significantly advanced kidney disease.* On the flip side, there are many people who *will* show signs of kidney disease. There are any number of symptoms that one can experience, so it is important to be alert to the changes noted below and to take the time to investigate what could be either a potential clue or sign of serious kidney damage.

WHAT ARE THE SIGNS AND SYMPTOMS OF KIDNEY DISEASE?

You know your own body better than any doctor. Therefore, it is important to pay attention to the signals it sends you. We will first briefly review the signs and symptoms that can be seen in kidney disease—the things you should be looking out for—and then focus on the blood work that can signal the presence of kidney disease. If you notice any of the following indications in yourself, get to a doctor to have it checked.

Proteinuria (Protein in the Urine) and/or Hematuria (Blood in the Urine)

One symptom of kidney disease that some people describe concerns changes in either the color or consistency of their urine. They may describe their urine as being frothy or bubbly, which can be a sign of protein leakage in the kidney. This is called *proteinuria (pro-teen-urea)* and is discussed more later in this chapter.

Others may notice tea- or dark-colored urine, or gross blood in the urine, which is called *hematuria (heem-a-turea)*. Hematuria can mean many things. If back pain is present, it can be a sign of a kidney stone or a kidney or bladder infection. It can also be a sign of a condition called *nephritis (neff-frye-tiss)*, in which specific types of inflammatory conditions that can affect the kidneys are present. While beyond the scope of this book, depending on your age and other health problems, hematuria can also be a symptom of cancer anywhere along the urinary tract. *Blood in the urine should never be ignored; see your doctor as soon as possible if it is happening to you.*

Problems with Urination

Men, especially those with an enlarged prostate, sometimes complain of difficulty with urine flow or maintaining a steady urinary stream. They may frequently make attempts to urinate throughout the night—a condition known as *nocturia (knock-turea)*. This can also be a symptom of kidney disease. If the prostate is grossly enlarged, it may partially or totally block the flow of urine and worsen kidney function. If this is happening to you, your doctor will likely refer you to a *urologist (your-ala-gist)*—a type of surgical doctor who specializes in problems of the entire urinary tract.

Women, on the other hand, sometimes describe burning with urination, or the need to constantly go to the bathroom. Such symptoms could mean either a bladder infection or early kidney infection. There are some young women who, in childhood or early teenage years, suffered from frequent urinary tract infections (UTIs). If you have a child or teenager with frequent UTIs (more than three to four a year), or if you are a young woman with recurrent UTIs, you should also consider seeing a urologist. Frequent UTIs could result from the bladder—which, remember, is the temporary holding tank for urine—not emptying completely, or it can mean a problem elsewhere in the urinary tract. A urologist can pinpoint where the problem is and begin to treat it. If, however, the problem is left untreated, it can affect kidney function over time.

Additionally, some patients—men and women—with diabetes may have trouble completely emptying their bladders. Urinary incontinence, often seen in elderly patients, is a common bladder-emptying problem. However, not all problems with urination mean you have a bladder problem. Some people with very advanced kidney disease complain of difficulty urinating or note a decrease in the amount of urine they make. If you notice any changes in your urinary habits, you need to call your doctor right away.

Edema

Some people may describe swelling in their legs, ankles, feet, hands, bellies, and/or around their eyes. This is called *edema (a-deema)*, and the extra fluid build-up can be a sign of significant kidney disease, as the kidneys are unable to rid the body of excess salt and water. Edema can also be a sign of excessive protein leakage by the kidneys into the urine—called proteinuria, as previously mentioned. The leakage of large amounts of protein into the urine can cause fluid to accumulate in the body, particularly in the legs. The fluid buildup can also cause a dramatic increase in body weight. Those affected may have difficulty putting on their shoes or buttoning their pants because of significant edema.

If you begin to notice any or all of the above symptoms in yourself or a loved one, call your doctor right away. Depending upon the cause of the edema, you may be referred to a kidney specialist.

Uremic Symptoms

If kidney function has worsened to the point that the kidneys are no longer working, patients may describe what doctors call *"uremic (your-ee-mick)* symptoms." When it has reached this level of severity, the kidneys can no longer filter and eliminate toxins. As a result, these substances accumulate in the blood, eventually reaching dangerous levels.

Uremic symptoms can include nausea, dry heaves, vomiting, excessive tiredness, lethargy, loss of appetite, loss of taste, food having a metallic taste, difficulty concentrating, abnormal sleeping patterns, hiccups, and/or severe itching all over without any other symptom. I have had several patients describe the last two symptoms as their only complaints. And sometimes, the only presenting symptom is something as subtle as, "I just don't feel right."

The important point is this: Many patients with kidney disease will *feel fine*. So again, at the bare minimum, I advocate for everyone to see their doctor at least once a year for an annual physical with blood work—even those people with no history or risk factors of kidney disease. I cannot emphasize enough the importance of reviewing your blood work with your doctor, as it is the *primary determining factor in diagnosing kidney disease.*

WHICH BLOOD AND URINE TESTS ARE USED?

When your primary care physician or kidney specialist, also called a *nephrologist (nef-ralla-gist)*, examines your blood work report, his or her primary concern is: *How well are your kidneys doing their filtering job?* The following tests and test results aid doctors in finding the answer.

Glomerular Filtration Rate (GFR)

If you recall, the small filters within the kidneys are called glomeruli. One important part of routine blood work reports is the Glomerular Filtration Rate, or GFR. The GFR is a calculated value and is an indication of how well the millions of glomeruli are working together, or at what rate and capacity your kidneys are filtering. This is the single most important piece of information your doctor needs, as it indicates the presence and severity of kidney disease.

Creatinine Level and Its Relation to the GFR

A common blood test your doctor may order is called the *creatinine (cre-a-ti-nine)*, and it provides a hint of what your kidney function may be. It is a separate kidney-specific blood test included in the routine blood work the doctor orders. Creatinine is a material made by your muscles and filtered by your kidneys. In general, the lower the creatinine number, the better the kidney function. Some doctors may look solely at this number as an indicator of kidney function. However, looking at the creatinine level alone is not enough to properly evaluate kidney function. In fact, the creatinine level is important only because it is used to calculate the GFR.

For the past several years, routine blood work has included a value calculation called an electronic GFR (eGFR). The lab automatically calculates the eGFR based on the creatinine level. The eGFR has proven invaluable in diagnosing kidney disease that otherwise would have been missed if a doctor had relied solely on the creatinine level.

Problems with Reliability of Creatinine Level

There are many things that affect the reliability of a creatinine level. Creatinine is dependent on a person's muscle size. For example, since men are typically more muscular then women, a creatinine of 1.0 mg/dl may represent normal kidney function in a man, but can suggest significant kidney dysfunction in a woman. Similarly, in a very muscular person or in someone with significant muscle loss due to certain medical conditions, the creatinine may not be a good indicator of kidney function.

In addition, certain commonly used medications, like Bactrim (trimethoprim-sulfamethoxazole) and Tricor (fenofibrate) used to treat high triglyceride levels, can affect the creatinine level, making it unreliable. The use of certain muscle-building supplements like creatine can also affect it. Your doctor should be aware of all medications, including over-the-counter and herbal supplements, you are taking.

Blood Urea Nitrogen (BUN)

Commonly obtained in routine blood work, the blood urea nitrogen (BUN) level is often used in combination with the creatinine level to alert doctors to changes in kidney function, particularly when the level changes from normal. When the BUN level is very high, it can be a sign of significant dehydration. This value can also be high in response to other conditions, as well. For example, some types of internal bleeding from the stomach or small intestine can cause a high BUN level.

Urinalysis

Your doctor may order a urine test, called a urinalysis, to further evaluate your kidneys. This is an important test that can signal early kidney disease by detecting abnormalities in the kidneys, even if your kidney function, as measured by the GFR, is normal.

To perform a urinalysis, your kidney doctor or primary care doctor will ask you for a urine sample, and then either do what's termed a urine dipstick test in the office, or send the urine sample to a lab. Several factors can be determined by the dipstick analysis including the presence of a UTI, the presence of glucose in the urine (usually a sign of diabetes), and the presence protein or blood in the urine (sometimes a sign of kidney inflammation called nephritis).

You may not notice any symptoms from the findings the dipstick test reveals. For instance, the amount of blood or protein in the urine may be so microscopic that it is invisible to the eye. That is the reason why many doctors will order a urinalysis—to detect these changes early. In my practice, as well as in many other kidney doctors' practices, the urine is further examined under a microscope for signs of infection or nephritis after the dipstick is obtained.

Quantifying the Amount of Protein in the Urine

The presence of protein in the urine as discovered through a urinalysis will likely prompt your doctor to order additional tests to better quantify the amount of protein you may be losing. This is discussed in detail in the following chapter. *Proteinuria (prot-een-or-eya) is the single most important predictor of worsening kidney function.* I can't overstate the importance of testing for this.

Other Blood Work

There are many causes of kidney disease, and once it is discovered that you have it, your primary care doctor or your kidney doctor will order more tests to get a better understanding of why your kidney function isn't normal. If your doctor determines that your kidney disease is more of a chronic nature, she will need to order additional blood work. This battery of blood and urine tests will give her a clear indication of your kidney function.

WHEN ARE IMAGING STUDIES NECESSARY?

If the results of your blood work suggest evidence of kidney disease, your doctor may order an ultrasound to get a visual picture of your kidneys. This non-invasive test can show if your kidneys are blocked or obstructed, as well as reveal kidney size and texture. There are findings on a kidney ultrasound that can indicate whether or not you may have chronic kidney disease. Further studies, such as a CAT scan or an MRI, play a role in diagnosing specific kidney conditions; however, each is not without its inherent risks. This is discussed in more detail in Chapter 7.

Kidney Early Evaluation Program (KEEP)

The National Kidney Foundation (NKF) is a valuable resource organization that provides doctors, patients, and their families with up-to-date information and education regarding kidney disease. In an attempt to detect and eradicate kidney disease in its earliest phases, the NKF has developed a program called the Kidney Early Evaluation Program (KEEP), which allows for comprehensive screenings to be performed at local sites. Check out the program's website at www.kidney.org/news/keep/index.cfm for further information.

SUMMARY

The kidneys are the body's filters and are responsible for keeping all the other bodily systems in balance. Certain blood and urine tests, including the GFR and the urinalysis, are invaluable in helping your doctor determine if a kidney problem exists. Understanding the signs and symptoms of kidney disease, listening to your own body, and effectively communicating changes to your doctor are all very important to your kidney and overall health.

2

Setting the Stage of Kidney Disease— Where Do You Stand?

Once you have been told you have kidney disease, the next step involves understanding the extent of your kidney damage. To help you, a CKD (chronic kidney disease) staging system was developed. This system describes the severity of kidney disease and also helps doctors assess its progression and prescribe specific treatment plans.

There are five stages of kidney disease—ranging from stage one to stage five—each of which represents a level of declining kidney function. Stages one and two are defined as mild kidney disease; stage three, as moderate kidney disease; and stages four and five, as advanced disease.

Each stage is based on the GFR—or filter—performance, measured in milliliters per minute (ml/min). Remember that the GFR (glomerular filtration rate) is important in evaluating how well your kidneys are functioning as filters. The five stages are explained in terms of approximate percentage of kidney function, which will give you a clearer understanding of the GFR values at each stage. All of the stages have their own distinguishing features. You and your doctor should discuss what exactly should be done at each in order to maintain and possibly improve kidney function.

STAGE ONE

In stage one, kidney function is normal or near normal—around 90 percent—but proteinuria is present. The GFR is greater than 90 ml/min. (Normal GFR is in the range of 100 to 130 ml/min.) Left untreated, this condition can lead to a worsening of kidney disease in the future. Remember that *protein in the urine is the single most important marker for predicting the future risk of worsening kidney function.*

The Importance of Proteinuria

On an average day, your kidneys will reabsorb about 99 percent of the protein that you eat. Normally, about 150 to 200 milligrams (mg) of protein are eliminated daily in our urine. If the amount of protein excreted is above this level, it can be an early sign of kidney damage.

Imagine your kidneys as fishing nets that filter and capture most of the protein you eat each day. Now picture someone taking scissors and cutting small slots in the net, allowing some of the protein to leak through the holes. When this happens, the kidneys become bombarded by excess protein. It increases their workload, creating a vicious cycle—the more protein the kidneys have to break down and remove, the more work the kidneys have to do. This causes irreversible damage; the kidneys get "scarred up" and their function can worsen over time.

Proteinuria commonly happens with diabetes-related kidney disease. There is also some compelling evidence that proteinuria not only causes damage to the kidneys, but also may be an early sign of vascular disease. Many heart doctors will order urinary protein levels routinely, as high levels may predict future heart disease, as well.

Ways of Measuring Urinary Protein Levels

There are two methods that can be used to measure the amount of protein in urine. The first is a random urine sample, which involves urinating into a plastic cup one time. It is usually done at a local testing center or lab, and in most instances, this testing will be sufficient. With this type of random test, the doctor will initially order the total amount of a special kind of urinary protein called albumin. This test is very sensitive and is a very early indicator of kidney disease. In addition, it may be an early predictor of future heart disease and vascular disease. If the levels of albumin in the urine, or *albuminuria (album-in-orea)*, are high, then the doctor will likely order another random urine sample to quantitate the total amount of protein in the urine. Under certain circumstances, however, your doctor may order a different type of urine test.

This second test consists of you urinating into a special plastic container every time you need to go over a twenty-four hour period. The lab will provide you with the container and directions to follow. There are two important tips to remember with this type of collection. First, plan to do it sometime when you will be home for the whole day. Second, the container needs to be kept cold, which is best done in the refrigerator. Before placing it in there, though, make sure you inform family members that its contents are not for drinking and keep it out of young children's reach.

The important point is this: *Proteinuria is serious. Levels higher than normal require more investigation and will usually require referral to a kidney specialist.*

STAGE TWO

I call this the "in-between stage." Kidney function is down to 60 to 89 percent of normal, and the GFR ranges from 60 to 89 ml/min. Compared with stage one, there is a decline in overall kidney function and proteinuria may or may not be present. At this early stage, close monitoring of your kidney function and a plan of action, which may include a consultation with a kidney specialist, should be initiated to prevent progression to the next stage.

STAGE THREE

This is the "turning point stage," because injury to the kidney beyond it is usually irreversible. Kidney function is 30 to 59 percent of normal and the GFR is 30 to 59 ml/min. At this stage, intervention by a kidney specialist is strongly recommended to delay the course of progression. If your primary care doctor has not already referred you to see a kidney specialist, he should do so now. Also at this stage, the eGFR on your blood work will report a specific value. (At stages one and two, the eGFR will only report >60 ml/min.) In stage three, other body systems are affected, as well, and you can begin to see changes in blood and bone health because of the advancement of kidney disease.

Blood Abnormalities

Remember that your kidneys make a hormone called *erythropoietin (erith-ro-po-eaten)*, which stimulates the body to make more red blood cells. At stage three of kidney disease, the kidneys may not produce enough of this hormone. When this happens, there is a risk of developing a low blood count, which is commonly called anemia. This condition is confirmed by a *hemoglobin (heme-o-glow-bin)*, or Hgb level blood test. As of this writing, an acceptable Hgb level for someone with CKD is between eleven and twelve. This accepted value, however, may change in the future as the guidelines are being re-evaluated.

Signs and symptoms of anemia can include fatigue, weakness, shortness of breath, and dizziness. If you experience any of these symptoms, call your doctor immediately. Also, note that people with certain conditions such as diabetes can have anemia even before reaching this stage; they may have a low Hgb level as early as stage one.

Bone Abnormalities

Bone health is maintained through the interaction of vitamin D, calcium, phosphorus, and a hormone called parathyroid hormone, or PTH. The kidneys' role in all of this is to transform vitamin D. This changed form of vitamin D regulates the amount of PTH made, which in turn regulates the amount of calcium and phosphorus needed by the bones. At this stage of kidney disease, vitamin D is not fully transformed; therefore, PTH goes unregulated, which can drastically affect bone health.

STAGE FOUR

Stage four represents the beginning of advanced kidney disease. Kidney function is 15 to 29 percent of normal, and the GFR is 15 to 29 ml/min. When you reach this stage, your kidney doctor will look for ways to maximize your remaining kidney function, as well as introduce a treatment plan that includes going for a transplant evaluation and preparing for dialysis.

In the best case scenario, you will already have a kidney doctor following you prior to this stage. Referral to a kidney specialist at this point is too late, because the kidney disease is so advanced that there is often little chance of improving kidney function. Unfortunately, time and again nephrologists are first consulted at this irreversible stage, but the window of opportunity to improve kidney function has already been lost.

Transplant Evaluation

When your kidney function is less than or equal to 20 percent (GFR < 20 ml/min), your kidney specialist will discuss referral to a dedicated transplant center for an evaluation. There is evidence that people do better when they are transplanted earlier, before dialysis is even started. Therefore, early intervention is encouraged because the transplant evaluation is a long process.

Transplant evaluation is important for determining eligibility for a kidney transplant. Factors such as age and the cause of your kidney disease are important considerations. Other medical conditions such as diabetes, heart and lung problems, and vascular disease are also important factors in determining if you are a suitable candidate.

As a potential transplant candidate, you will undergo thorough, lengthy evaluations by a transplant surgeon, a transplant nephrologist, or another member of the transplant team. Additional physicians, including heart doctors (cardiologists) and other medical sub-specialists are also involved in the evaluation process as needed. Sometimes, if there has been a change in one of your other medical conditions or if you are ill, the evaluation process is temporarily put on hold.

When the testing is complete, you will be placed on a transplant waiting list if you are approved. Family members or close friends can then be tested to determine if they are able to donate a kidney to you. This is strongly encouraged, as, given the shortage of available kidneys, a person could be on the list for a long time.

Dialysis

At this advanced stage, you will most likely be informed about dialysis, including the various options and types, of which there are several. Dialysis is not actually needed at this stage, but there is so much that goes into its preparation that beginning to talk about it is recommended.

Dialysis is an "artificial filtering process" that does the job the kidneys are no longer able to do. Hemodialysis (HD) is the most common type. With it, you are connected to an HD machine that filters, cleanses, and returns your blood through an access. There are several types of accesses, including a catheter and a graft, but the best type of access is called a *fistula (fis-chu-la)*. A fistula is created by a vascular surgeon, usually in the non-dominant arm—the one you don't write with or use often. A well-functioning fistula allows you to get an excellent dialysis treatment. After surgery, it can take two to four months before a fistula can be used.

Because of the amount of time it takes—including the evaluation by the vascular surgeon, the surgery itself, as well as the time it takes for the fistula to mature—the kidney specialist will begin discussing this very important preparatory step at stage four.

An HD treatment is usually three to four hours long, and occurs three times a week. You can decide on a schedule to accommodate your lifestyle. There are even a couple of newer options from which to choose. One includes nocturnal dialysis, which involves doing dialysis overnight three times a week at dedicated "nocturnal units." And more recently, *home* hemodialysis is becoming an increasingly popular alternative. Here, after a few weeks of training, you are doing a similar type of dialysis at home using a small, portable HD unit. You and a partner of your choice—it is recommended to train someone else, as well, but not necessary—are essentially doing what the nurse or technician does at the dialysis unit. There is great flexibility with home HD; on average, a person will do four to five treatments a week for two to three hours at a time.

Another type of dialysis is called *peritoneal (perry-toe-neil)* dialysis (PD). This involves a special kind of catheter that is placed in your belly by a surgeon. A series of exchanges is then performed throughout the day. With each exchange, the belly is filled with about two liters (two quarts) of a glucose-based fluid. There is then a "dwell period" where the fluid remains in the belly and the dialysis "is being done." Each dwell period can last anywhere from two to four hours. The fluid is then drained from the catheter. An advantage of this type of dialysis is that it can be done at home. However, many people find it hard to get used to the idea of carrying fluid around in the belly.

Alternatively, PD exchanges can be done by an automated system where the exchanges are done at night via a machine called a cycler. If a person has had multiple surgeries in his belly, he may not be a candidate for PD. Like home HD, PD requires several weeks of training, usually done by a dedicated dialysis nurse along with your doctor. See the Resources section (page 161) for access to more information about PD.

All of this information can be overwhelming for patients to digest. For that reason, I prefer to discuss this life-altering process over two or three visits with family members present whenever possible. I have provided several websites and other references relating to dialysis in the Resources section (page 161) for your convenience. Dialysis is a bridge to transplantation for many patients. It is important to get evaluated as soon as you are able, while considering all of your options.

STAGE FIVE

At this final stage of kidney disease, kidney function is less than 15 percent and the GFR is less than 15 ml/min. At this point, you may or may not be undergoing dialysis treatment. Dialysis is usually started when kidney function is less than 10 percent (or GFR < 10 ml/min), although people with diabetes-related kidney disease may be started when their kidney function is 15 percent or less (or GFR < 15 ml/min). As with most things, however, there are exceptions to this rule.

In certain circumstances, if you are feeling good and not experiencing any of the uremic symptoms discussed earlier, dialysis may be postponed; however, your blood work will still be followed closely by your doctor and he will likely ask you to follow up with frequent office visits. Similarly, if you are on the cusp of starting dialysis you will be monitored closely with frequent follow-up visits.

SUMMARY

The stages of chronic kidney disease are indicators of your kidney function. At each stage, the goal is to work with your doctor to maximize kidney function and prevent progression to the next stage. You should vigilantly review your blood work with your doctor, and when applicable, be referred to a kidney specialist. Your kidney health depends on it.

3

$\mathcal{I}$nteracting with Healthcare Professionals

The healthcare system is highly specialized and complex. Having been diagnosed with kidney disease, you are probably dealing with several different healthcare providers. Given the sheer number of doctors and practitioners, it is important that a smooth, coordinated system of care is provided to you. The goal of this chapter is to clarify the duties of the healthcare providers with whom you will likely interact, as well as to discuss the important role you play in your own healthcare team. This chapter will also provide you with tools that will enable you to maximize visits with your kidney doctor.

THE TEAM MEMBERS

There are several important members of your healthcare team. I use the team concept to explain the various members, and to describe how they *should* interrelate with you and with one another. The team members should include a primary care doctor, a kidney specialist, a nutritionist, a case manager, physician extenders, other specialists, complementary health providers, and you, the patient. All of these members play different but valuable roles in your healthcare.

Primary Care Doctor

When you are experiencing a health problem, the first individual you seek out is your primary care doctor. Therefore, she is often the first to identify a problem with your kidneys. Most primary care practitioners are either board certified or board eligible in family practice or internal medicine. You should feel comfortable with your primary care physician, and your relationship should be based on mutual trust and respect.

Kidney Specialist (Nephrologist)

When your primary care doctor suspects a kidney problem, she will often refer you to a kidney specialist, or *nephrologist (nef-ralla-gist)*. Nephrologists have training in internal medicine, as well as additional training in kidney disease and hypertension, specifically. Your kidney doctor should be board eligible or board certified in nephrology.

Depending on your stage of kidney disease, you will likely be following up with your kidney doctor on a regular basis, so your relationship with her is one of the most important you will develop. Generally, the more advanced the stage of kidney disease, the more frequently you will be asked to follow up with your doctor. If you are at stage four or five, you are likely seeing your kidney doctor more often than your other healthcare providers.

Nutritionist

Good nutrition is essential for maintaining health, especially if you have kidney disease. Making the right food choices and understanding the role of proper nutrition is important. Many people have more than one complex medical problem, including diabetes, hypertension, or heart failure. In these instances, a consultation with a nutritionist is essential; unfortunately, the ability to obtain this consult in our managed care environment is often difficult.

In the outpatient setting, it can be difficult to secure a visit with a dietitian unless you have diabetes and advanced kidney disease.

Even if you can, you have to pay out of pocket. This can be expensive, especially if continued monitoring and follow-up is needed. If you have stage five kidney disease and your doctor starts you on dialysis, you will be receiving feedback from the nutritionist frequently—at least on a monthly basis if not more. While the feedback at this stage is invaluable, it is somewhat ironic because if it had been done sooner, it may have had a greater impact.

Case Manager

If you have stage five kidney disease and are starting dialysis, you will be interacting with a social worker or case manager. This integral team member helps you navigate the complex insurance issues that often arise at this stage. With rare exceptions, patients in the earlier stages do not interact with case managers.

Physician Extenders

Physician extender is a term used by doctors and other health professionals to define two kinds of healthcare providers—nurse practitioners and physician assistants. Physician extenders work closely with a supervising doctor and provide invaluable help. Some people are hesitant to see physician extenders. You always have a choice in whom you wish to see; however, with the shortage of doctors, especially kidney specialists, physician extenders are important in providing care. Depending on where they work, their duties can vary. The focus here will be on their potential roles in a nephrologist's practice.

Nurse Practitioner (NP)

The nurse practitioner has earned a bachelors degree in nursing, and has an additional graduate degree. Working with a kidney doctor, she can see patients in the office or hospital setting, order blood work and other tests, and prescribe treatment, including medication.

Physician Assistants (PA)

The physician assistant has obtained a bachelors degree, usually in a health sciences related field but this can vary, with additional graduate training resulting in a masters degree. The range of care offered by the PA is similar to that of the NP. You will likely encounter both the NP and PA in many physician practices and hospitals.

Other Specialists

Depending on the cause of your kidney disease, you will likely be seeing other specialty doctors. For example, if you have diabetes and diabetes-related kidney disease, you will probably see an *endocrinologist (endo-krin-ala-gist)*, or blood-sugar specialist. And if you have heart problems, then you are likely following up with a *cardiologist (kar-dee-alla-gist)*, or heart doctor.

Complementary Health Providers

Other members of your health care team may include practitioners of complementary medicine, including homeopathy, natural medicine, massage therapy, acupuncture, and others. Certain complementary treatments or supplements can interact with prescribed medication and may influence kidney function. Therefore, there should be open communication between you, your kidney specialist, and your complementary health providers. The key is to take full advantage of all of your healthcare providers' skills to ensure a coordinated plan of care.

You, the Patient

As the patient, you are the most valuable player on your healthcare team; you are the captain of the ship, so to speak. The job of the other team members is to inform and empower you to make the best treatment decisions possible. You, however, are ultimately responsible for your own health.

THE TEAM RULES

As with any team, there are rules that need to be followed in order for it to be successful. The most important rule is communication.

Your health care team members need to communicate respectfully and effectively with you and with each other.

The most common method of communication is through paper correspondence. After an office visit, some health providers may write down a visit summary; others may choose to talk into a tape recorder or other recording device, and then have their notes transcribed onto paper.

Regardless of the recording method, visit summaries often include an assessment of your medical condition and plan of care. Copies are either faxed or mailed to each of your healthcare providers. Depending on the nature of the visit, telephone communication may sometimes be needed.

CKD CLINICS

Comprehensive CKD clinics are becoming popular with patients and doctors alike. These fantastic clinics allow for frequent follow-up office visits, especially for patients in the advanced stages of CKD, where more coordinated and structured care is needed. Another benefit of these clinics is that they allow various members of patients' healthcare teams to come together, which facilitates communication.

CKD clinics can take many forms, depending on the specific office practice. In many cases, the physician extender works closely with you and your kidney doctor for more frequent follow-up care. For example, if you have advanced CKD, you may visit with your kidney specialist every two to three months, although this can vary. In between visits with her, you may be seen more frequently by a physician extender. Depending on your particular situation, you may also be seen by a nutritionist or a case manager, if needed. This is good for continuity, and many people do better with this "team approach" to care.

HOW TO MAXIMIZE AN OFFICE VISIT
WITH YOUR KIDNEY DOCTOR

Being healthy, especially concerning kidney health, is not a passive process. It is important that you are an active member in the process. One example of this is knowing how to get the best out of your doctor visits. Doing so involves two steps. The first is preparing for the visit, and the second is the actual visit itself. The following information is geared towards visits with your kidney specialist specifically, but this process can and should be used with all of your healthcare providers.

Preparing for an Office Visit

Preparing for an office visit involves performing some of your own background checks. There are different ways of evaluating if a doctor may be the right fit for you, even before your first scheduled visit. For instance, you may know some friends or family members who can give you their opinions of the doctor. There are also websites you can go to, such as www.healthgrades.com, where you can see how the doctor is rated. For additional resources, please refer to page 161.

Many people are apprehensive the first time they are told they need to see a kidney doctor. When scheduling an initial visit with one, make sure she gives you enough time; in my practice, new patients are given an hour for their first visit. To prepare, write down a list of any questions you have and bring it with you. You should also bring a list of all of the medications you are taking, including dosages. Be sure to add any vitamins, herbs, supplements, and over-the-counter medications, as well, as everything you take matters.

During an Office Visit

Your office visits should be organized and efficient. Here is a checklist of what you should do during your appointments to maximize your time:

- If possible, bring a friend or family member with you. They can be a great source of support, ask questions you may not have even thought of, and provide comfort during visits.

- Be specific about any signs or symptoms you may have. Examples include those previously mentioned in Chapter 1, including difficulty with urination or edema.

- Review your blood work with your doctor. Nephrology is a lab-based specialty, and it is important to understand your blood test results. Ask specifically about the GFR level, blood count, potassium level, and urine studies.

- Always get copies of your blood work and maintain your own file.

- Pay attention to the blood pressure obtained in the office, so that you can correlate it to what your readings have been at home. (Hint, hint. As we will discuss, it is important to take your blood pressure at home.)

- Bring a pad and pencil, and write down everything the doctor says in terms of prescribed treatment. Make sure it makes sense to you.

- Ask any questions you have regarding prescribed treatment, especially medication. If something is prescribed, ask if it is brand name or generic. With blood pressure medication, for example, there may be a difference between the efficacy of the generic medication and the brand name. Also ask about what side effects you should look out for.

You should feel comfortable during the visit with your kidney doctor. If you do not, seek out other health professionals until you find one that meets your needs. *Remember, your doctors work for you.*

SUMMARY

The relationship between you and your team of healthcare specialists is special. Adequate "face time" with your doctors is important in helping you make the best treatment decisions possible. Remember that you are responsible for your own healthcare. Your doctors and other healthcare providers can help you and give informed decisions; however, it is important to take an active role in your own kidney health, as it is ultimately in your hands. *You are the MVP of your team.*

PART TWO

Inflammation, Causes of Kidney Disease, and Standard Treatments

In Part Two, our goal is to focus on the nitty-gritty of kidney disease. There are many different causes of kidney disease but they do have certain things in common, including the fact that many are also causes of inflammation. The future study of kidney disease will be a study of inflammation—not only researching the many ways that the kidneys are affected by inflammation, but also discovering how inflammation can affect (i.e., damage) other organs of the body, including the heart.

In order to begin to better understand the inflammation process, we have to start small—very small. Heck, we need to get microscopic to the level of the cell. The cell of any organ is the basic unit of life, and in Chapter 4 we look at the study of the kidney by first looking at the cell. This is where the inflammatory process begins, but it can easily become a never-ending cycle as inflammation will only cause further inflammation and damage.

In Chapter 5, we begin to look at the most common medical conditions that can affect the kidneys. Many of the conditions discussed, including hypertension, diabetes, and obesity, are already epidemics themselves and continue to spread like wildfire. In reading this chapter, I urge you to keep this important thought in mind: hypertension, diabetes, obesity, and vascular problems that affect the kidneys are themselves inflammatory conditions. The keys to stopping this cycle of inflammation are aggressive early intervention and prevention.

In Chapter 6, we look at what I call the high-level inflammatory syndromes, as well as a common inherited condition called polycystic kidney disease. We will also examine important causes of kidney dysfunction, particularly in older men, that can block or obstruct the urine flow.

Chapter 7 is very important because it focuses on side effects of commonly prescribed medications as well as the potential effects of commonly ordered imaging procedures. Before taking any medication or undergoing any procedure, you will learn the right questions to ask including: *What are the effects of this medication or procedure on my kidney health and what are the alternatives?*

And finally, in Chapter 8 you will read about the various ways that the body is affected by kidney disease. From your blood to your bones to your heart to your cells, kidney disease has far-reaching effects. You will gain some insight into these important effects, as well as an understanding regarding your treatment options.

4

$\mathcal{T}$he Inflammatory Response, Oxidative Stress, and the Kidneys

The goal of this chapter is to think about kidney disease and the conditions that can affect kidney function in a very different way. Why is this so important? Because as doctors and scientists study kidney disease, they are learning about the significance of *inflammation*; they are finding that it plays a major role in worsening kidney disease.

Inflammatory changes in the kidneys are not caused only by medical conditions that affect kidney function, but also by the kidneys themselves. This chapter focuses on the following three important themes:

- Chronic kidney disease itself is a state of inflammation.

- The conditions that cause chronic kidney disease, such as hypertension, diabetes, and obesity, are themselves inflammatory conditions and should be thought of as such.

- The inflammation of kidney disease is not limited to the kidneys; it can affect other organs as well, specifically the heart. A vicious cycle ensues where worsening kidney function can affect heart function and vice versa.

The current research and future treatment of kidney disease will involve not only treating the specific condition affecting the kidneys, but also managing and reducing the associated inflammatory component as well. Therapies aimed at preventing progression of CKD will be focused on how to reduce the level of inflammation affecting the kidneys. In order to understand how to reduce the inflammatory response, we need to first review what inflammation is and what stimulates the inflammatory response.

INFLAMMATION AND OXIDATIVE STRESS

Inflammation is basically how the body normally responds to any type of illness, disease, or trauma. A cut in the skin, for example, sets in motion a rapid inflammatory response. The body immediately makes proteins called *cytokines (site-o-kynes)* that begin the healing process. Over time, a scar made of strong fiber-type tissue will form to protect and minimize further injury to the site. This is what the body is supposed to do—work to heal itself.

What if, however, the injury was inside of you and you couldn't see it? For example, what if there was ongoing scar formation going in the kidneys that you couldn't see or feel? What if the inflammatory response was never really turned off? How would such a process get started? The answer to this last question is something called *oxidative stress*. Oxidative stress refers to damage that is occurring inside the cells of your body. It is this continued stress within the cells that stimulates and perpetuates the body's inflammatory response.

The body is designed to maintain harmony and balance, especially at the cellular level. The cell is the tiniest, most basic unit of life. Each cell performs its tasks in perfect harmony with the body's other cells. Knowing this is important because *oxidative stress and inflammation begin at the cellular level.*

Our cells normally exist in a natural or "reduced" state. Any disturbance in the natural state of the cell causes the production of toxic materials called free radicals. Examples of disturbances could include any type of illness or injury. When this happens, our cells make antioxidants whose job is to stabilize the cells and "defuse" these toxic oxygen radicals. But the more free radicals that are

Transforming Growth Factor (TFG)-Beta

Remember the question that was asked: *What if there is ongoing scar formation going on in your kidneys that you can't see or feel?* In particular, scar formation is the end result of a cytokine called transforming growth factor (TGF)-beta. TGF-beta is associated with scar-like tissue formation inside the body called *fibrosis (fy-bro-siss)*. Fibrosis, like scars, is permanent and irreversible. TGF-beta is implicated in the worsening of diabetes-related kidney disease, other kidney conditions, and chronic kidney disease itself, all of which are *states of chronic inflammation*. There is ongoing research regarding this particular cytokine.

formed, the more damage that is caused to the cell. If the disturbance to the cell is continuous and severe enough, too many free radicals are formed and the damage to the cell is significant. The cells themselves become "oxidized," which means the checks and balances within the cells deteriorate, and individual cells are no longer able to effectively repair the damage.

As this cellular domino effect happens, the body's inflammatory response is over-stimulated. These toxic oxygen radicals are catalysts for even more inflammation. Cytokines, or pro-inflammatory proteins, are produced. Examples of these include *endothelin (en-doe-thiel-ien)*, interleukins, and transforming growth factor (TGF)-beta. Many cytokines can go on to produce chronic inflammatory changes in the body, including scarring that begins at a microscopic level.

Several conditions, such as diabetes, hypertension, *glomerulonephritis (glom-are-ulo-nef-ritis)*, *nephrotic (nef-rot-ik)* syndrome, and CKD itself, can cause oxidative stress to the cells and are potent stimulators of the inflammatory response. This can lead to scarring of the kidneys because the inflammatory response is never really turned off. Therefore, treating the underlying condition affecting the kidneys will ultimately preserve kidney function and decrease the level of inflammation.

OTHER CAUSES OF INFLAMMATION THAT CAN AFFECT THE KIDNEYS

In addition to certain medical conditions, there are other circumstances that can activate a similar inflammatory response in the kidneys. These include occupational and environmental exposures, as well as dietary factors. Laboratory research suggests that toxic exposures could perhaps be inherited and passed on from one generation to the next.

Environmental and Occupational Exposures

From the air we breathe to the water we drink, our bodies are exposed to multiple toxins on a daily basis that can affect our kidney health. Additionally, certain occupational exposures to heavy metals like cadmium, lead, mercury, uranium, and others, as well as hydrocarbons related to certain types of industrial manufacturing, can cause kidney disease. Heavy metal toxicity of the kidneys causes continuous oxidative stress, subsequent inflammation, and worsening of kidney function over time. The effects of heavy metals on kidney function, especially lead, is discussed in detail in Part Three of this book.

Dietary Factors

There is strong evidence showing that the cause of some kidney diseases, specifically nephritis and the nephrotic syndrome, may result from an inflammatory reaction due to allergens in the processed foods that we eat. This is discussed in greater detail in Chapter 6, which is about immune-related syndromes. In addition, the low antioxidant value of the food we consume may also have a contributory effect.

Prior Toxin Exposures

An interesting study performed by Dr. Michael Skinner and his research group at Washington State University examined the question: Could a medical condition that a person has now be a consequence of a past generation toxin exposure during pregnancy? It is a known fact that many drugs and toxins can affect the kidney function of a developing fetus early in a pregnancy.

In this animal-based study, Dr. Skinner and his group found that conditions such as kidney disease and disorders of the immune systems were the effects of a toxin that continued through four consecutive generations. Essentially, it suggests that a toxin exposure from past generations could play a role in developing kidney disease, as well as many other diseases, in future generations. This was only a single study, but it does raise some important questions that require further study.

THE EFFECTS OF INFLAMMATION ON THE BODY

Up until this point, we have been focusing specifically on inflammation as it affects the kidneys. It is important to remember that because the body functions as an interconnected unit, the inflammation affects the body as a whole. Thus, the risk of *atherosclerosis (ath-iro-sklair-osis)* and peripheral arterial disease (PAD) is dramatically increased in CKD.

In CKD, inflammation can become a vicious, never-ending cycle. There is evidence to suggest that regardless of the cause of kidney disease, CKD is itself a potent inflammatory condition. The inflammation from CKD has a toxic and life-altering effect on the heart; it increases the risk of heart disease and can shorten one's lifespan. The damaging effects of inflammation on the heart and kidneys have been described in a condition called the cardio-renal syndrome.

In this syndrome, problems with the heart can cause a worsening of kidney function. The reverse of this is also true—worsening kidney function has been implicated in heart problems, including coronary artery disease and congestive heart failure (CHF). In many instances, it is difficult to determine which organ is the primary culprit; most likely a sizeable inflammatory response causes failure in both organs. Significant heart and kidney problems, characterized by congestive heart failure, hypertension, and worsening kidney function, make this syndrome very difficult to treat.

RENIN-ANGIOTENSIN-ALDOSTERONE SYSTEM (RAA SYSTEM)

As previously mentioned in Part One, the hormones made by the kidneys and adrenal glands help regulate blood pressure. Unfortunately, they are also hugely responsible for thrusting the kidneys' inflammatory response into overdrive, especially in cases where high blood pressure, diabetes, or various forms of nephritis are involved. One of the mainstays of CKD treatment, no matter the cause, has been the use of certain classes of blood pressure medications that block the RAA system. These medications, called ACE inhibitors and angiotensins receptor blockers—or ARBs for short—can reduce the level of inflammation in the kidneys and help preserve kidney function. They may also reduce the level of TGF-beta, which was discussed earlier. In addition, these same medications have a heart-protective effect. They are fully discussed in the following chapter.

PREVENTING THE INFLAMMATION PROCESS

I do not want you leaving this chapter thinking that in regards to inflammation, all is lost and nothing can be done. This is completely untrue. In fact, the inflammatory effects of many of the conditions that can cause CKD, including hypertension and diabetes, can be minimized or even prevented. All it requires is a commitment to change your life and lifestyle. As you will read in the forthcoming chapters—especially Part Three—changes that promote a healthier lifestyle including exercise and dietary modification can reduce the inflammatory load and help prevent progression of CKD. There are many other things that you can do to help your kidney health and reduce the inflammatory response, as well. Again, this is discussed in detail in Part Three of this book.

SUMMARY

Kidney disease is an inflammatory condition that can have detrimental effects on your health—especially your heart health—and can shorten your lifespan. What's important is that once you know you have this condition, there are things you can do to assist your body in stopping the inflammatory response. By changing your lifestyle and your diet, you can help prevent inflammation and many of the conditions that you will be reading about in the coming chapters.

5

Common Causes of Kidney Disease

In this chapter, we will explore in detail the medical conditions frequently responsible for causing CKD, some of which were briefly mentioned in earlier chapters. Diabetes and hypertension remain the two most common—and in many ways most preventable—causes of kidney disease in this country. Over thirty percent of our population is obese, and obesity is also a very common, yet under-recognized cause of kidney disease. In our aging population, vascular disease, or atherosclerosis, is becoming a more recognized cause of kidney disease. As you read through this chapter keep in mind one important point: While diabetes, hypertension, obesity, and vascular disease are individual conditions, they can and often do frequently occur together.

DIABETES

Diabetes mellitus, commonly called just *diabetes*, is a devastating medical condition that can affect the eyes, nerves, nervous system, blood vessels, heart, and kidneys. There are two different types of diabetes: type 1 and type 2. In type 1 diabetes, the body does not make insulin. Most people are diagnosed with type 1 diabetes at a young age, and many may develop problems with the blood vessels in their eyes, which is called *retinopathy (retin-a-pathie)*. If left untreated, their vision can worsen. In type 2 diabetes, the body is able to make insulin, but the insulin doesn't work like it is supposed to. Because of obesity and other factors, the body develops a resistance to it.

When diabetes leads to kidney disease, it is called diabetic *nephropathy (nef-ra-pathie)*. About one fourth of those diagnosed with type 1 diabetes will go on to develop kidney disease, and many of them will also have retinopathy. About ten percent of those with type 2 diabetes will go on to develop kidney disease, although this may be a low estimation. Diabetic nephropathy is the most common cause of kidney disease in this country, and the number of people diagnosed is skyrocketing as more and more of our younger generation is being affected.

How Diabetes Effects the Kidneys

Diabetes strains the kidneys and increases their workload, which causes inflammatory changes. Over time, these changes can contribute to scarring and a worsening of kidney function. There are many ways that diabetes can affect the kidneys. Let's take a look at them, starting with proteinuria, which is the main way the kidneys are impacted by diabetes.

Proteinuria

If you remember, proteinuria is the single most reliable predictor of worsening kidney function. In diabetes, doctors watch the protein levels in the urine closely. They will often order a special type of urine protein test called albumin, because it is a very good indicator of early kidney damage. Measured in milligrams (mg), a level less than 30 is considered normal. If you have between 30 and 300 mg of albumin in the urine, your doctor will likely start treatment involving the use of certain medications and lifestyle changes. If you have more than 300 mg of albumin in your urine, *referral to a nephrologist is strongly recommended.* In addition, diabetes and proteinuria can affect the integrity of the blood vessels, increasing inflammation and the risk of atherosclerosis in the kidney, heart, and a number of other organs of the body.

High Blood Sugar, High Blood Pressure, and Obesity

In addition to proteinuria, high glucose (blood sugar) levels can also increase the stress and workload on the kidneys. This is why tight control of blood sugars is so important. Many people with diabetes, especially type 2, also have high blood pressure and are obese, both of which can also contribute to a worsening of kidney function.

The RAA System

Diabetic nephropathy affects the kidneys through the effects of the RAA system. As mentioned in Chapter 4, the hormones in this system regulate blood pressure and are also responsible for increasing the inflammatory response in the kidneys. By increasing the activity of cytokines like TGF-beta, the RAA system can worsen proteinuria and increase scarring and fibrosis in the kidneys. This is why I believe that diabetes is an inflammatory condition, and the RAA system is an important contributor to this inflammatory process.

The Angiotensin Converting Enzyme (ACE) Gene

There is evidence that genes—or DNA—can influence how our bodies are affected by states like diabetes. A certain gene called the angiotensin converting enzyme, or ACE, may in part determine the degree to which the kidneys are affected. Variations in this gene may significantly contribute to the differences concerning the extent of kidney damage and proteinuria in different people with diabetes.

The ACE gene is being researched for other medical conditions, as well, not just those involving the kidneys. In the future, knowing one's genetic makeup will likely guide treatment for diabetic nephropathy and other medical conditions.

Standard Treatment Approaches

There are many things you can do to improve your kidney health as it relates to the impact diabetes has on it. Lifestyle changes—including weight loss, exercise, and dietary modification—are the most important, and are discussed in detail in Part Three. The focus here is on the standard treatment approaches used in the treatment of diabetic nephropathy, which will, in turn, support kidney health.

Tight Control of Blood Sugars

Diabetes is diagnosed when your fasting blood sugar (glucose) level is greater than 126 mg/dl as measured on two different occasions. If your blood sugars are high, your doctor will likely prescribe lifestyle changes as previously mentioned, and if needed, medications whose job is to help control your blood sugars. In certain cases, your doctor may need to prescribe insulin.

There are many different classes of medications used to treat diabetes. As with all medications, it is important to talk with your doctor about the correct dosing and possible side effects of each. If your blood sugar levels are still not controlled with lifestyle and medication changes, a consultation with an endocrinologist—a doctor who specializes in diabetes—is needed.

Tight Control of Blood Pressure

Tight control of blood pressure is important, even if proteinuria is not present. The current recommendations aim for a blood pressure reading of less than 130/80 if no proteinuria is present. If proteinuria is present, the blood pressure goal is lowered to 125/75. These are just general guidelines, however.

In diabetic nephropathy, where higher than normal blood pressure often accompanies diabetes, it can be difficult in some people to maintain a top blood pressure number in the low 120s and a bottom number in the low to mid 70s. In addition to advocating lifestyle changes, your doctor may need to prescribe additional medications to lower the blood pressure. You will likely be asked to monitor your blood pressures at home; you should get into the habit of doing so if you are not already.

Use of ACE Inhibitors or ARBs

In addition to lowering blood pressure, these two classes of medications also protect the kidneys, as they can reduce protein levels in the urine. Angiotensin converting enzyme (ACE) inhibitors and angiotension receptor blockers (ARBs) work by blocking different aspects of the RAA system. In doing so, they lessen the inflammatory response.

Examples of ACE inhibitors include lisinopril (Zestril), enalapril (Vasotec), and ramipril (Altace). Examples of commonly used ARBs include olmesartan (Benicar), valsartan (Diovan), telmisartan (Micardis) and irbesartan (Avapro).

If your doctor prescribes a medication from either of these two classes, it is important to be aware of possible side effects. For instance, ACE inhibitors can cause a hacking type cough, which can occur any time after the medication is started. In a very small percentage of people, ACE inhibitors can cause a life-threatening reaction called *angioedema (angie-o-edema)*, a type of allergic reaction which causes swelling of the tongue or vocal cords. If it happens to you, stop the medication and call your doctor or 911 immediately.

Another possible side effect of ACE inhibitors and ARBs is an increased potassium level. About one week after taking the medication, blood work should be done to check the potassium level and monitor kidney function. A very high potassium level can affect the heart, so this needs to be watched closely. Some people with diabetes normally have higher-than-normal potassium levels, because diabetes can affect the kidneys' ability to rid the body of excess potassium. If that is the case, you may not be able to take medications from either of these two classes.

If you are unable to take an ACE Inhibitor or ARB, there are other prescribed medications that can decrease protein levels. A class of medications called the aldosterone antagonists—spironolactone (Aldactone) and eplerenone (Inspra)—has been shown to reduce protein levels. Another medication called aliskiren (Tekturna) has shown a decrease in proteinuria in those who took it over a six-month period. Other medications that can reduce protein levels are verapamil (Calan) and diltiazem (Cardizem), members of a class of blood pressure medications called calcium channel blockers.

These classes of medications will be discussed further in the next section concerning hypertension. With them, your blood pressure, potassium level, and kidney function need to be closely watched, and you need to be aware of all of their side effects. A common side effect of spironolactone (Aldactone) is breast tenderness, which may require either reducing the dose or stopping the medication entirely. The calcium channel blockers listed here won't affect potassium levels. As medications in this class can slow your heart rate, your doctor will be watching your blood pressure and pulse carefully to be sure they don't drop too much.

Tight Control of Cholesterol and Triglycerides

High cholesterol and triglyceride levels can affect kidney function through their effects on oxidative stress and worsening inflammation. Lowering these levels can help improve kidney function and overall health. In addition to lifestyle changes that can lower cholesterol and triglyceride levels—such as changing to more of a vegetable-based diet and exercising (see Part Three)—commonly prescribed medication classes include fibrates, which lower triglyceride levels, and statins, which lower the "bad" or LDL cholesterol. Statins may also reduce protein levels and are thought to have an anti-inflammatory effect, as well.

Examples of statins include atorvastatin (Lipitor) and simvastatin (Zocor). The fibrates include fenofibrate (Tricor).

Blood work that monitors liver function needs to be done frequently after starting medication from either of these two classes. Call your doctor immediately if you develop unexplained pain or cramping in your arms or legs, as it may be secondary to these medications. An uncommon reaction in the form of muscle damage due to the medications called *rhabdomyolysis (rab-doe-myo-lyciss)* can develop; if severe enough, it can cause kidney failure. Statins can affect memory, and you should be aware of this, as well.

There are some great books published by Square One Publishers concerning options for lowering cholesterol, including *Natural Alternatives to Lipitor, Zocor, & Other Statin Drugs*. See the Resources section (page 161) for references regarding these natural alternatives. But be sure to talk with your doctor before starting any medication to make sure it is okay to take with kidney disease. Concerning statins, pay attention to the dosage your doctor prescribes. Many of the side effects discussed above are seen with higher dosages, and dosage adjustments may need to be made if kidney disease is present.

HYPERTENSION

Hypertension, or high blood pressure, is often referred to as the silent killer. It is the second most common cause of kidney disease in this country, and a leading cause among African Americans. Hypertension affects many organs of the body, including the heart, brain, blood vessels, and kidneys.

Blood pressure measurements that are obtained in the doctor's office are used as an initial guide to determine how severe your blood pressure is. As you may be aware, the top number on the blood pressure is referred to as the *systolic (siss-tollik)* blood pressure. The bottom number is called the *diastolic (dye-a-stollic)* blood pressure. While doctors do pay attention to the lower number, it is the top number—the systolic blood pressure—that really increases the risk of heart disease, stroke, and kidney disease, especially as we get older. Your doctor will ask you to take your blood pressure at home and record it, as well, because for many patients, being in the doctor's office can cause a rapid elevation in the blood pressure numbers, termed "white-coat syndrome."

How Hypertension Affects the Kidneys

The kidneys and other body organs are designed to handle blood pressures within a normal range. If the pressure delivered to them stays high over a prolonged period of time, it can have harmful effects on the body's systems. For example, heart disease and congestive heart failure are long-term consequences of uncontrolled high blood pressure. In the brain, hypertension is an important risk factor for stroke.

The kidneys also do not tolerate the stress of high blood pressure. Uncontrolled high blood pressure causes inflammatory changes in the blood vessels. Over time, the arteries begin to become *sclerosed (skler-ost)* or scarred, which is called *atherosclerosis*. Left unchecked

The Different Stages of Hypertension

As you may know from visits to the doctor's office or from surfing the Internet, there are different stages of hypertension, depending on blood pressure level. In 2003, a group of expert panelists and physicians basically redefined hypertension and emphasized a focus on early treatment and management even before high blood pressure is diagnosed. The *Seventh Report of the Joint National Committee on Prevention, Detection, Evaluation, and Treatment of High Blood Pressure* (commonly referred to as JNC 7) were, in my opinion, ingenious in defining the new classes of high blood pressure.

A normal blood pressure is now defined as a systolic blood pressure (the top number) of 120 or less, and/or a diastolic blood pressure (the lower number) of 70 or less. The next stage, which is called prehypertension, is defined by a systolic blood pressure of 120 to 139 and/or a diastolic blood pressure of 80 to 89. This stage is very important, because it is an excellent time to not only adopt lifestyle changes that reduce the risk of developing hypertension, but also to focus on other risk factors that may be present, including diabetes or prediabetes, obesity, high cholesterol levels, a smoking habit, a sedentary lifestyle, and poor dietary habits. It is no surprise that all of those factors are risk factors for worsening kidney disease, as well; nor is it a surprise that many of the conditions occur together.

In this new classification scheme, there are two stages of hypertension, stage 1 and stage 2. Stage 1 defines a systolic blood pressure as 140 to 159 and/or a diastolic blood pressure of 90 to 99. In stage 2, the systolic blood pressure is 160 or higher and/or the diastolic 100 or higher. Antihypertensive medication is usually prescribed at this stage. If you have stage 2 hypertension, two or more medications may be needed.

and untreated, hypertension can cause *fibrosis*—irreversible scarring—to the kidneys.

Standard Treatment Approaches

Lifestyle changes are the most important changes you can make for your kidney—and your own—health. By exercising, stopping smoking, lowering the amount of sodium in your diet, and losing weight (if needed), you can lower your systolic and diastolic blood pressures, perhaps without even needing to take any medication in the first place. These are very real things that you can do that can help maintain and improve your kidney health, and these changes will be discussed in detail in Part Three.

There are also many classes of medication that your doctor may choose from in treating hypertension. The following information includes key points regarding a few classes of blood pressure medication. Talk with your doctors regarding your treatment options. The listing below should only serve as a generalized treatment guide.

Use of ACE Inhibitors or ARBs

In addition to lowering blood pressure, ACE inhibitors and ARBs are beneficial for both the kidneys and the heart. Many doctors will first choose a medication from these two classes. If a patient of mine had CKD, I would need a significant reason not to prescribe an ACE inhibitor or ARB given their protective effects.

One of these significant reasons is potassium level. If someone has high potassium levels, she will not be able to take these medications. In someone with advanced kidney disease (stage 4 or stage 5), using these medications is like having a double-edged sword. While there are studies that show they can delay the worsening of kidney function *over time,* any stress on the kidneys—any type of serious illness, for example—can worsen kidney disease in the presence of either of these two classes of medications. There is also an increased risk of higher potassium levels. Close monitoring of your kidney function and potassium levels are required if you are placed on one of these medications.

If the above factors are absent and someone has both diabetes and hypertension, then these are the recommended classes of medications to begin treatment with.

Use of Calcium Channel Blockers

In addition to reducing blood pressure, calcium channel blockers also have other beneficial effects. For instance, amlodipine (Norvasc), one of the most studied medications, helps protect the heart and reduces the risk of stroke. A major article has changed how many doctors are using it to treat hypertension. If after first using either an ACE inhibitor or an ARB the blood pressure remains high, amlodipine (Norvasc) has been found to be a good second choice option. If you have proteinuria, your doctor may instead choose either diltiazem (Cardizem) or verapamil (Calan), as either of them can be used in conjunction with an ACE inhibitor or ARB to reduce protein levels.

Examples of medications prescribed from the calcium channel blocker class of medications include amlodipine (Norvasc), nifedipine (Procardia), felodipine (Plendil), and isradipine (DynaCirc). Moreover, diltiazem (Cardizem) and verapamil (Calan) not only reduce protein levels, but they are also used by heart doctors for the treatment of certain types of *arrythmia (a-rith-mia)*, or abnormal beating of the heart, because they can slow the heart rate.

The main side effects of these medications include constipation and edema. Some patients may also complain of a mild headache.

Use of Diuretics

In addition to lowering blood pressure, *diuretics (dye-er-etiks)* are used in the treatment of edema and congestive heart failure. There are several different classes of diuretics—Thiazide, Loop, and Potassium-sparing—each of which have their own unique uses.

Thiazide diuretics include hydrochlorothiazide (Diuril) and chlorthalidone (Thalitone). They can be used by themselves or in combination with ACE inhibitors and ARBs for a more potent effect on lowering blood pressure. Thiazide diuretics are less effective in advanced stages of kidney disease. Their main side effects can include low sodium, potassium, and magnesium levels. In addition, it can elevate uric acid levels in some patients. If you have gout, be careful when taking a Thiazide diuretic. Moreover, they may also cause dehydration. Call your doctor if you feel dizzy or lightheaded as this can be a sign that your blood pressure may be too low.

Loop diuretics include furosemide (Lasix), bumetanide (Bumex), and torsemide (Demadex). They are used more for the treatment of edema that can be seen in the higher stages of chronic kidney disease, though they can have modest effects on blood pressure. The main side effects can include low potassium and magnesium levels. When on a loop diuretic, your doctor may have you obtain blood work on a frequent basis and will ask you to weigh yourself daily. If you experience a significant change in your weight—either gaining or losing too much—over a day or two, it will require a change in dosage of your medication. Again, call your doctor if you feel dizzy or lightheaded as this can be a sign that your blood pressure may be too low.

Finally, potassium-sparing diuretics can raise potassium levels. They need to be used carefully in advanced stages of CKD (GFR < 30 ml/min), as the risk of high potassium can hinder their use. Potassium-sparing diuretics include spironolactone (Aldactone), eplerenone (Inspra), amiloride (Midamor), and triamterene. All of them can reduce proteinuria, and spironalactone (Aldactone) and eplerenone (Inspra) are also used in the treatment of heart failure. In addition to high potassium levels, if you are taking spironolactone (Aldactone), a significant side effect is breast and nipple tenderness. This requires decreasing or even totally stopping the medication for the symptoms to disappear. As with all diuretics and blood pressure medications, call your doctor if you feel dizzy or light-headed as this can be a sign that your blood pressure may be too low.

Use of Renin Inhibitors

Renin inhibitors represent the first new class of blood pressure medication in years. They work by blocking the effects of renin. The only medication in this class is aliskiren (Tekturna). It can also lower urine protein levels, as documented in one study. One common side effect is high potassium. Since it has only been out for a very short time, its long-term effects need to be studied further.

Use of Beta Blockers

This class of medications is used to lower blood pressure, and has found its niche in those who have suffered a heart attack and those with congestive heart failure. Examples of medications prescribed from this class include metoprolol (Lopresor), atenolol (Tenormin), and nebivolol (Bystolic). Nebivolol (Bystolic) represents a newer class of beta blockers.

Beta blockers can sometimes slow the heart rate, so it is important to take your pulse in addition to monitoring your blood pressure. If your heart rate is less than fifty-five, notify your doctor as he may need to make medicine or dosing changes. Other side effects can include fatigue, weakness, depression, and problems with libido. Call your doctor if you experience any of the above symptoms.

Use of Alpha Blockers

Alpha blockers lower blood pressure and are commonly used in men with enlarged prostates, as they can help improve urine flow and stream. Examples of medications prescribed from this class include doxazosin (Cardura) and terazosin (Hytrin).

Alpha blockers can cause significant dizziness when standing up, specifically when first starting the medication; be careful and stand up slowly when taking this medication. If you have significant light-headedness or dizziness, call your doctor right away.

In addition to the many classes of medications used for blood pressure that were just described, there are also others. When talking to your doctor about them, it is important that you ask about their possible side effects and safety in kidney disease.

Medication Combinations

The average person takes several different medications. In an effort to reduce the pill burden and increase compliance with medications, there have been many single pill combinations created. One example is a combination of both valsartan and hydrochlorothiazide called Diovan HCT. Other examples include a combination of amlodipine and benazepril called Lotrel, and a combination of olmesartan and amlodipine called Azor. In the last two examples, an ACE inhibitor or ARB is combined with a calcium channel blocker. These are very popular combinations often used by physicians.

There is both an upside and a downside to combination medications. If the blood pressure is very high and very difficult to bring down, which can happen in the setting of CKD, then two or more medications are often needed. While using a combination medication decreases the quantity of pills someone has to take, if there is a reaction to a medication, it can be difficult to know which of the two medications is the culprit. Also, giving two medications together may be too much at one time for some people. If your doctor suggests that you begin taking a combination medication, be sure to ask him about possible side effects as well as interaction with other medications you may be taking.

Screening for Resistant Hypertension

Despite being on a several different medications, it may be difficult to get your blood pressure under control. If "white-coat syndrome"—high blood pressure in the doctor's office but normal at home—is not present, then other causes need to be investigated. These can include kidney disease, obesity, vascular disease (problems with blood vessels) of the kidney, and sleep apnea. Note that there are many other causes of high blood pressure; your doctor may have started investigating these causes, or may have consulted a kidney specialist for further treatment and evaluation.

OBESITY

Obesity is a common cause of hypertension and kidney disease. It is estimated that over 30 percent of the people in this country are obese. The definition of obesity is actually a mathematical calculation that your doctor does during an office visit: It is your weight divided by your height, squared. This calculation determines what is called your body mass index, or BMI. Obesity is defined as a BMI greater than 30.

In addition to the toll that excess weight has on total body health, it can wreak havoc on the kidneys. It is often seen in combination with both diabetes and hypertension, and the damaging effects that all three can have on the kidneys is incredible.

How Obesity Affects the Kidneys

Obesity is a state of inflammation and is a direct risk factor in and of itself for worsening kidney disease, even in the absence of hypertension and diabetes. Like hypertension and diabetes, it can cause an inflammatory response in the kidneys.

Obesity and High Blood Pressure

Increased weight is a strain on the heart and the kidneys. It can raise blood pressure and stimulate the RAA system that has been mentioned multiple times in this book. Obesity is also linked to sleep apnea, which is another unrecognized cause of resistant high blood pressure. Sleep apnea is covered in detail in Part Three of this book.

Obesity and the Metabolic Syndrome

The combination of a BMI greater than 30, high fasting blood sugar levels, high triglycerides, and uncontrolled blood pressure is called the metabolic syndrome. The increased weight causes resistance to the actions of insulin in the body. This common syndrome increases the risk of developing diabetes, kidney disease, heart disease, stroke, and vascular disease. Weight reduction and lifestyle modification are the gold standards of treatment.

Obesity and Proteinuria

There is a direct link between obesity and proteinuria, even in the absence of diabetes. Increases in proteinuria correspond to increases in weight. There is also a condition called obesity-induced *glomerulopathy (glo-mare-u-la-pathy)*, where the stress on the kidneys is so great that it can cause them to lose significant amounts of protein in the urine. This condition is often reversible and usually resolves with weight loss.

Standard Treatment Approaches

Lifestyle modifications are the most important way to change your life, lose weight, and improve both your overall health and your kidney health. This is so important that it will be discussed separately in Part Three.

There are also certain medications that are used in the treatment of obesity. For more information regarding them, I strongly suggest opening a dialog with your doctor. When I have obese patients with kidney disease, I try strongly to encourage lifestyle modification first and foremost.

Finally, for those whose weight is significant and very difficult to lose, your doctor may suggest *bariatric (bare-e-at-rick)* surgery as a means to lose weight. It is an option for many people, but as with any procedure, you need to make sure it is right for you. You should do some preparation work on your own and ask the right questions before your doctor visit.

VASCULAR DISEASE

As people are living longer, vascular disease, or atherosclerosis, and its role in kidney disease is becoming a more recognized problem, especially in the older population. It is commonly seen in people with hypertension and diabetes, because they can often have problems with the blood circulation in other parts of their bodies. Many will have coronary artery (heart) disease or problems with blood flow to the legs, called peripheral arterial disease, or PAD. There may also be problems with the blood circulation in the *carotid (car-rot-tid)* arteries in the neck, which can increase the risk of stroke. The treatment of problems with blood flow to the kidneys, however, is very individualized given the complex issues involved.

Think of the *aorta (eh-orta)*, the largest artery in the body, like the trunk of a huge tree. Responsible for supplying blood to the entire body, it has many branches that travel throughout. A small, single branch off each side of the tree trunk goes to both kidneys. The narrowing of any artery can affect the blood flow to the kidney, which is called *stenosis (ste-nose-sis)*. There are a couple of ways that the artery to the kidneys can become stenosed (narrowed); the most common cause is atherosclerosis to the artery, or plaque buildup that occurs over years. States of inflammation can quicken this process, as it can for any blood vessel in the body.

How Vascular Disease Affects the Kidneys

Vascular disease, or atherosclerosis, is a process that occurs over several years. If the plaque level builds up in the artery to such a degree that the narrowing is significant, the kidneys may not receive the blood they need and the kidney function can be affected. When this happens, many people will feel and appear perfectly normal. Some, however, may show certain signs and symptoms due to the significant narrowing in the artery.

One such sign is blood pressure that just won't stay down. If you are on more than three medications for high blood pressure and your doctor is having a difficult time regulating it, he may begin to suspect that there is a problem with the blood flow to your kidneys. Another sign is recurrent heart failure. If you have developed a buildup of fluid in your lungs and your doctor says your heart is fine, he may suspect that you have problems with the blood flow to your kidneys.

After starting on an ACE inhibitor, your doctor may ask you to have follow-up blood work done a week or so later. If your kidney function suddenly gets worse or if your potassium level increases, that can also be a tip-off that you have problems with the circulation to your kidneys.

Those at Risk for Vascular Disease in the Kidneys

Patients with diabetes are at a higher risk for vascular disease in the kidneys. Those with evidence of circulation problems in other areas of the body—carotid, coronary, or peripheral vascular disease—are also at risk. In addition, elevated *homocysteine (homo-sis-teen)* levels may increase the risk of developing vascular disease. Homocysteine is an amino acid, and it is thought that high levels in the blood may be a risk factor for atherosclerosis. This can be measured by a simple blood test. High cholesterol and high triglycerides are also risk factors. Inflammation also can increase the rate of atherosclerosis. Your doctor may order a blood test called a *sedimentation (said-duh-men-*

tashe-un) rate, or he may choose to order a C-reactive protein, because they can indicate the level of inflammation in the body.

Standard Treatment Approaches

The initial evaluation and management of vascular disease of the kidney still remains somewhat of a gray area. There are several different options concerning imaging studies to better look at the blood flow to the kidneys. Each type of study, as you will see, is not without its limitations or potential adverse effects. Likewise, the treatment for severe stenosis is not without its potential problems. The treatment plan is often individualized for each person, depending on age, signs and symptoms present, other medical conditions, and viability of the kidneys.

Diagnostic: Imaging Studies Your Doctor May Order

If your doctor suspects a problem with the blood flow to your kidneys, she may order a special type of ultrasound, called a Doppler ultrasound. This commonly ordered imaging test can give an indication of how well the blood is flowing to your kidneys. If the Doppler ultrasound suggests that there is a significant narrowing of the artery, then your doctor may opt to order another type of imaging test, including an MRI or a special type of CAT scan.

If you have an increased BMI, your doctor may suggest obtaining an MRI or a CAT scan as a first line imaging study, as the Doppler ultrasound may not provide enough diagnostic information. These studies are not without their inherent risks, which are dealt with in detail in Chapter 7. Your doctor may also refer you to a vascular surgeon for a consultation.

Treatment: Medical Options

If it is discovered that the stenosis of the artery is significant—more than 70 percent of the artery is blocked—your doctor will discuss treatment options. These may include medications and supplements, as well as dietary and lifestyle changes, to aggressively reduce the factors for atherosclerosis. As stated, this involves minimizing the risk factors of atherosclerosis. Common standard therapy includes

The Angiogram

One imaging procedure that was not mentioned before is the angiogram. Although it is considered by doctors—including nephrologists and vascular surgeons—to be the "gold standard" in diagnosing stenosis of occluded vessels like the arteries going to the kidney, it is not without its risk.

Often, determining the right imaging procedure is an involved discussion involving the patient, her family, and her family doctor, kidney doctor, and vascular surgeon. The pros of an angiogram include direct visualization into the artery of the kidney, with the ability to also treat the affected area in one procedure. The contrast dye used can affect the kidneys, but the amount of dye used can be minimal. The cons of an angiogram, on the other hand, include the fact that it is an invasive procedure, and that if an intervention is done, there can be complications to that procedure (see forthcoming section on angioplasty and stenting).

lifestyle modification and dietary changes. Your doctor will be checking your cholesterol profile and will be very aggressive in treatment. Tight control of blood pressure and blood sugars is very important, as is lowering of homocysteine levels and promoting a lower level of inflammation in the body. (Yes, this can be done!) This will be discussed in detail in Part Three.

Treatment: Procedural Options

In addition to medical treatment, your doctor will likely also talk to you about performing a more invasive type of procedure if the stenosis to the artery is significant. This type of procedure first involves performing an angiogram as described above. Then, after the narrowed area is visualized, an *angioplasty (angie-o-plas-tie),* or opening up the narrowed area with a small balloon, is followed by the placement of a stent, or small tube to make sure the narrowed area stays open. Given the possible complications of this invasive procedure, it has not been promoted as a routine practice, with each situation carefully scrutinized and evaluated before any treatment is done.

Complications: Difficulties with Angioplasty and Stenting

If you remember, atherosclerosis refers to a plaque buildup that occurs along the walls of the blood vessels—a process that takes years. During the angioplasty, a process called *embolization (em-bole-is-zation)* can occur. Here, a small piece or pieces of plaque can break off as a result of the balloon angioplasty. These small emboli can travel to smaller arteries of the kidneys and cause an acute inflammatory reaction. This can affect kidney function, and it is not an uncommon complication.

If the kidney function is advanced, it is often not clear-cut whether or not to proceed with the angioplasty. In some cases, placement of the stent may not improve the renal function. Given the risks of the procedure, most physicians will only consider this procedure in one of two situations: first, if the blood pressure is dangerously high despite multiple medications, and second, if there is only one functioning kidney and the blood flow to that kidney is severely compromised. There is an ongoing study that is looking at medical versus invasive treatment, and the results of this should be completed over the next few years. I tend to take a very conservative approach and only recommend an invasive approach when there are no other options.

SUMMARY

There is a common theme that began in the last chapter and is continued on in this chapter; it is the dangerous effects of inflammation on the kidneys. Hypertension, diabetes, obesity, and atherosclerosis often occur together. The damaging effects of these four inflammatory conditions on the kidneys can worsen kidney function. Prevention in the forms of weight loss, lifestyle changes, and dietary improvements are important to preserve your kidney function. There are also standard treatment options, including medications and procedures, but they are not without their possible side effects; sometimes the treatments are even worse than the disease itself, so be sure to always maintain an open dialog with your doctor.

6

Other Conditions That Can Affect the Kidneys

In addition to diabetes, hypertension, obesity, and vascular disease, which were discussed in the previous chapter, there are other conditions that affect the kidneys and impact a person's quality of life. This chapter focuses on the high-level inflammatory syndromes, polycystic kidney disease, and the management of conditions that can block the flow of urine and prevent the kidneys from emptying completely.

THE HIGH-LEVEL INFLAMMATORY SYNDROMES

By now, you should be starting to understand the significant role that inflammation plays in kidney disease. There may be a difference, however, in the levels of inflammation associated with certain conditions. Different diseases can have different levels of inflammation. For example, cancer is associated with a very high level of inflammation. Certain kinds of infections and conditions like lupus and rheumatoid arthritis can also have very high levels of inflammation.

The conditions discussed here, *glomerulonephritis (glo-mair-ulo-ne-fry-tis)*, or GN, *vasculitis (Vas-q-ly-tis)*, and the *nephrotic (nef-ra-tik)* syndrome, or NS, can be associated with very high levels of inflammation, as well. One characteristic of these conditions is that treating them often requires the use medications that can radically affect the immune system. For example, chemotherapy is often used to treat cancer. Chemotherapy-like medications that can "lower" the immune system response are often used to treat the debilitating forms of lupus and rheumatoid arthritis. Similar medications may be used for bad cases of GN, vasculitis, and NS; these can also affect the immune system.

All three of these conditions are general categories that refer to a large group of many different conditions. This section focuses on general principles concerning diagnosis and treatment.

Glomerulonephritis (GN)

If you recall, the *glomerulus (glo-mare-ul-iss)* is a tiny system of blood vessels and very small arteries that work as filtering units for the kidneys. Glomerulonephritis (GN) refers to any condition that causes inflammation of these blood vessels. The degree of inflammation can range from mild to severe. Sometimes, depending on what is causing the GN, other body systems can also be affected.

In GNs mildest forms, there can be hematuria or proteinuria with little or only mild changes in kidney function. In its most severe form, people can have major hematuria or proteinuria, with very bad kidney disease (a very low GFR). They may also have edema and very high blood pressure. Many people will fall somewhere in between.

In children and young adults, IgA nephropathy and *post-streptococcal* (strep-toe-kakkol) glomerulonephritis (PSGN) represent the most common types of GN seen. The latter can occur several weeks after a child has "strep throat." PSGN usually gets better on its own after several weeks with no extra treatment, and the kidney function stays normal or near normal. In adults, examples of GN again include IgA nephropathy and GN related to lupus—with other organs being affected. Depending on the person, their symptoms, and the result of blood and urine tests, your doctor may need to prescribe the types of medications mentioned earlier.

Vasculitis

Vasculitis refers to other conditions that can cause inflammation of the kidneys' blood vessels. As with GN, the inflammation can be limited to the kidneys or involve other body systems, as well. Examples include Wegener's (Weg- a- nur's) disease, in which the sinuses and lungs can be affected, and Goodpasture's syndrome, in which the lungs can also be affected.

Nephrotic Syndrome (NS)

In the Nephrotic Syndrome (NS), a person will have significant proteinuria, but hematuria is usually not present. Another possible symptom is significant edema. There can also be abnormal blood work, including high cholesterol and triglyceride levels, as well as low protein levels in the blood. The low blood protein levels occur because the patient is losing so much protein in the urine (over three thousand milligrams of protein, with a normal amount being about 200 mg or less!). The body then begins to overproduce cholesterol, which is no longer being dissolved and transported properly through the system due to the lack of protein.

In children, the most common cause of NS is called minimal change disease. In adults, common causes include focal segmental *glomerulosclerosis (glo-mare-ulo-sklare-osis)* (FSGS) and membranous nephropathy. Understand that there are many causes of GN, vasculitis, and NS, and that there can be significant overlap among the three.

Diagnosis

The nature of the symptoms in conjunction with abnormalities in the blood and urine tests helps to determine the level of diagnosis and treatment. For example, if a person has normal kidney function and the protein levels in the urine are mildly above normal, your doctor will discuss closely monitoring your kidney function, as well as recommending lifestyle and dietary changes. If the condition should change, as in worsening kidney function or higher levels of proteinuria, your doctor will often recommend a kidney biopsy to help determine the type of process occurring.

The kidney biopsy procedure is usually performed by a nephrologist or interventional radiologist—a type of doctor who does this type of procedure quite frequently. The kidney biopsy is not surgery and is commonly done in the radiology department. The sample that is required is roughly the same size as the white part of your fingernail. The whole procedure takes roughly twenty minutes and will be fully explained to you. After the sample is obtained, it will be sent to a pathologist who specializes in kidney disease, who will then examine the biopsy specimen under a microscope to determine the process of inflammation. This procedure's risks include bleeding, so you will be asked to stay in the hospital overnight for observation.

Causes of the Inflammation

What causes the inflammation in these disorders? What is the trigger that predisposes the kidney to be the recipient of these high-level inflammatory syndromes? Why are some people more inclined than others to get this? Part of the answer to these complex questions may be as simple as the food choices we make.

We can all develop allergies to the foods that we eat. In some people, these food allergies can trigger a significant inflammatory reaction in the kidneys causing either GN or NS. A prevalent example is an allergy to gluten, which is a common ingredient in many types of bread, including wheat and rye. A gluten allergy can cause an inflammatory process in your stomach and intestines called celiac disease. Having celiac disease increases your risk of developing any form of nephritis or nephrotic syndrome. There have been several cases reported of either NS or GN in people who had celiac disease. The advent of gluten free foods has been a blessing to those with this syndrome.

In another study, adults diagnosed with NS who ate a low-allergy diet had a dramatic reduction in proteinuria. Moreover, in a study focusing on children who had been diagnosed with NS, there was a dramatic reduction in proteinuria when cow's milk was removed from the diet. And many of the children's urine protein levels remained low in follow-up. There are other reported cases where just by changing the nature of their diets, patients with other types of GN like IgA nephropathy were able to maintain kidney function and reduce proteinuria.

So what does this information suggest? It hints that there may be something in the food we are eating that is triggering nephritis or NS. But is it the preservatives, the food additives, or the coloring? Is the way the food is prepared? Or, is it a residual effect of how the farm animals are raised? Unfortunately, it isn't yet clear but hopefully will be sometime soon.

The information in these studies also suggests that one initial method of treating these conditions should be a low-allergy, inflammatory-free diet. It also suggests that figuring out what food allergies are present may be of benefit. Why certain people are more affected than others, however, remains a mystery.

Standard Treatment Approaches

The severity of kidney disease and the amount of protein in the urine will determine the degree of treatment. For those patients with mild disease—minimal proteinuria and normal or near-normal kidney function—your kidney doctor will likely monitor you closely. She will be asking you to obtain blood work on a routine basis to watch your kidney function, as well as for a urine test to follow your protein levels. In addition, she will prescribe either an ACE Inhibitor or ARB for its protein-reducing properties, and will closely follow your blood pressure and cholesterol levels. If you have significant edema, especially in your legs, your doctor may start you on a diuretic like furosemide (Lasix) to help with the swelling.

If your kidney function is abnormal or you are spilling a significant amount of protein in your urine, your doctor will likely talk with you about starting treatment with medications that can affect your immune system. This includes the use of medication such as prednisone, cyclosporine (Neoral, Sandimmune, or Gengraf), cyclophosphamide (Cytoxan), and mycophenolic acid (Cellcept). These medications are not without side effects. Some of them, including cyclosporine (Neoral, Sandimmune, or Gengraf) and mycophenolic acid (Cellcept), are also used for those who have undergone an organ transplant and need them to suppress their immune systems in order to prevent rejection. You need to speak with your kidney doctor at length regarding the benefits and risks of initiating such treatment. If your kidney function has been severely affected by the inflammatory process (GFR < 10 ml/min), you may also be asked to start dialysis.

POLYCYSTIC KIDNEY DISEASE

Polycystic kidney disease is usually referred to as *autosomal (auto-zo-mull)* dominant polycystic kidney disease, or ADPKD. Autosomal refers to how the condition is inherited; it is passed down from one generation to the next, and a family member has a 50 percent chance of developing it. In ADPKD, many fluid-filled sacs called cysts are found in the kidneys; some cysts can be located in the liver, as well.

There are two types of ADPKD. The first type, referred to as PKD1, is thought to be a more aggressive form of the condition. Those with PKD1 are thought to progress to end-stage kidney disease faster than those with PKD2. That being said, as the cellular and molecular mechanisms of ADPKD are being researched, there may be significant genetic variance in PKD1.

ADPKD is one of the most common inherited conditions responsible for kidney disease and patients needing to start dialysis. There is a significant amount of research going on as to the possible reasons that cysts form in the first place. I cannot say enough of the significant role and support of the PKD Foundation in educating and advocating for this disease.

How the Kidneys are Affected

In ADPKD, the cysts can grow so large they begin to overwhelm the kidneys. As they get larger, the cysts can compress and squeeze the kidneys, as well as increase the size of the kidneys. High blood pressure can be a problem as the cysts continue to get bigger.

The tremendous advances in science have made it possible for complex diseases like ADPKD to be better understood. It is possible to see what may be going on inside the cell, and it has been discovered that there are abnormalities in the cells themselves. Specifically, abnormalities in a protein called *aquaporin (aqua-pore-in)* have been identified and they will likely play a significant role in future treatment.

Standard Diagnostic and Treatment Approaches

Specialized genetic testing remains the best way to diagnose ADPKD. In people younger than thirty years of age, doing a kidney ultrasound to look for cysts is not recommended, as it is less sensitive for picking up cysts. If you have a family history of ADPKD, you should speak with your doctor about undergoing genetic testing or further imaging studies.

The mainstay of treatment involves tight control of blood pressure. The use of ACE inhibitors and ARBs, when tolerated, is recommended. There is nothing as of yet that will diminish the size of the cysts, but as previously discussed, I believe it is only a matter of time before a treatment is discovered.

A small percentage of people with ADPKD can develop aneurysms in the brain called Berry aneurysms. If a family member has had a history of brain aneurysm, then it is recommended that imaging be done to evaluate further. The most common imaging procedure recommended for this is a study called Magnetic Resonance Angiography (MRA). As will be discussed in Chapter 7, it is important to know the kidney function before going for this study.

Right now, there is no definitive treatment for ADPKD. There are some exciting things coming down the pipeline, however. The goal is tight control of blood pressure, which can be difficult as the cysts get bigger and further squeeze the kidneys. When the person's GFR approaches 20 percent, appropriate referrals are made to begin the transplant evaluation and the person is advised regarding dialysis options. Please refer to the reference section for other resources regarding ADPKD.

BLOCKAGE OF THE KIDNEYS

If you remember, the kidneys are connected to two tubes called ureters that empty into a large holding tank called the bladder. When the bladder is full, it triggers a reflex for it to empty. The urine then flows through a small tube called the urethra and out of the body. The kidneys, ureter, and bladder together are called the urinary tract. In older men, an enlarged prostate is a leading cause of an obstruction, or blockage, of the urinary tract, referred to as obstructive uropathy. Obstructed or blocked kidneys are a significant cause of kidney disease in older men.

How the Kidneys Are Affected

The extent that the kidneys are affected depends on the time and severity of the blockage. If there is little or no emptying of urine over time, the kidney function will be compromised. The longer the kidneys stay obstructed, the less likely that the kidney function will return to normal.

As many men get older, they develop difficulties with urination. The most common cause of this can be benign prostatic hyperplasia (BPH), especially in men over the age of fifty-five. The prostate is linked to the bladder like a ball to a glove; when the prostate gets larger it can block the flow of urine from the bladder. BPH is the most common cause of kidney obstruction in men.

Often, men will complain of difficulty starting urination, of often having to get up at night to urinate, and of the need to urinate frequently. If both kidneys are blocked, they may have trouble going at all. Conversely, there may be *no symptoms* at all, especially if only one kidney is affected.

Standard Diagnosis and Treatment Approaches

The simplest test that your doctor will order if she suspects kidney blockage is an ultrasound of the kidneys. The majority of the time, it will show an enlarged kidney, which is a sign of a blocked kidney. At this time, your doctor will most likely ask you to see a urologist—a doctor who specializes in the "plumbing" of the kidneys. The urologist will often ask you to undergo another, more comprehensive test such as a CAT scan or MRI to get a better picture of the blockage.

Once the diagnosis of an obstructed kidney is made, the urologist will likely need to do more invasive studies to determine the cause of the obstruction and alleviate the symptoms. If the cause is due to an enlarged prostate, then there are different options the urologist will discuss with you. The necessity of an invasive procedure will be determined by the degree of prostate enlargement. There are other procedures that may be performed by the urologist, but that is beyond the scope of this chapter.

SUMMARY

In kidney disease, it is important that doctors begin to think outside the box with regards to standard medical treatments. Nephrotic syndrome and glomerulonephritis are two examples of when this proves beneficial. Lifestyle changes, such as the avoidance of high-allergy foods and the use of a low-allergen diet, helps reduce proteinuria in many cases. This is not to say that standard treatment doesn't have its place, but dietary modification is an important part of the therapy.

If you have kidney disease, a kidney ultrasound should be part of the diagnostic work-up. In many cases, you may never know you have an obstructive process affecting the kidneys unless your doctors look for it.

7

$\mathscr{M}$edications, Imaging Studies, and Interventions

You have now learned about several different classes of medications, specifically those that lower blood pressure and reduce proteinuria. Yet under certain circumstances, these same medications can be harmful to the kidneys. Other classes of prescribed medication can also affect kidney function, including anti-inflammatory drugs, antibiotics, and medications used for the treatment of ulcers and gastroesophageal reflux (GERD). Moreover, certain over-the-counter medications such as ibuprofen and acetaminophen can also affect kidney function.

Some standard treatments can trigger an inflammatory reaction in the kidneys, and some can "stun" the kidneys. This chapter examines the possible effects and risks that certain imaging studies and procedures, as well as medications, have on kidney function.

MEDICATIONS THAT CAN INFLAME THE KIDNEYS

Certain classes of medications can cause a type of nephritis, or inflammatory response, in the kidneys. In the last chapter, we discussed one type of nephritis in detail. The focus of this section is another type called *interstitial (inter-sti-shull)* nephritis. Here, the inflammatory response is not directed against the glomerulus, but other areas of the kidneys. In this section, we will examine certain classes of medications that can cause this type of reaction in the kidneys.

Antibiotics

Antibiotics are extremely popular and are very commonly prescribed. Certain classes of antibiotics, including pencillins such as amoxicillin (Trimox); and a closely related drug class called *cephalosporins (cef-ello-spor-ins)* such as cephalexin (Keflex) and cef-uroxime (Ceftin) can cause interstitial nephritis in certain individuals. Trimethoprim-sulfamethoxozole (Bactrim) is usually prescribed for urinary tract infections and can cause this reaction, as well. In fact, any class of antibiotics can cause this type of inflammatory reaction, not just those described above.

Non-Steroidal Anti-Inflammatory Drugs (NSAIDS)

This class of medications, including the over-the-counter brands Motrin and Advil, as well as the prescription brands Celebrex and Naprosyn, can also induce a similar type of inflammatory reaction in the kidneys. Sometimes this reaction can be accompanied by a dramatic increase in proteinuria.

There is an irony here; these medications are used to treat a variety of inflammatory conditions like arthritis, but they themselves can stimulate an inflammatory reaction in the kidneys. Because of their side-effect profile, especially concerning the kidneys, you should be careful in using this class of medication. We will be talking more about NSAIDS later, as they can affect the kidney function in multiple ways.

Proton-Pump Inhibitors (PPI)

PPIs are used to treat ulcers of the stomach and small intestine, as well as to treat gastroesophogeal reflux disease (usually referred to as GERD). Examples include pantoprazole (Protonix) and esomeprazole (Nexium). Commonly prescribed for people both in and out of the hospital, PPIs can cause an inflammatory reaction in the kidneys, even after the medication has been taken for a while.

Bisphosphonates

The *bisphosphonates (biss-phos-pho-nates)* refer to a class of medications used to treat osteoporosis. They are also commonly used in people with cancer. Here I am referring to medications that need to be given through a vein, including pamidronate sodium (Aredia) and zole-dronic acid (Zometa). Pamidronate sodium (Aredia) can trigger a type of inflammatory reaction causing the nephrotic syndrome and worsening kidney function. Zoledronic acid can also worsen kidney function. The usage and dosing of both medications need close mon-itoring if kidney disease is present.

MEDICATIONS THAT CAN "STUN" THE KIDNEYS

In certain situations, medications that are normally beneficial and kidney protective can actually worsen the kidney function. Here is a common scenario that doctors often see:

Your dad (or mom) calls and tells you he is feeling weak. He may have had either a recent cold or "viral bug" accompanied by nausea, vomiting, or diarrhea, or some combination of the three. He hasn't had much of an appetite over the last several days, yet he has still taken all of his medications faithfully. He may have diabetes, hyper-tension, heart disease, or congestive heart failure, all of which are very common conditions in the older population.

Regarding his medications, he has been taking an ACE inhibitor and is also on a diuretic, such as furosemide (Lasix). He may also have significant arthritis, and despite his doctor's warnings he has been taking ibuprofen, more so when the weather changes and he notices his arthritis acting up more.

Concerned, you visit and notice that he is very weak and debili-tated. You call 911 or take him to the hospital yourself. You're now in the emergency room of your local hospital. Your dad had some blood work done, and the next thing you know you are being told by the emergency room doctor that his "kidneys are bad" and that a kidney doctor will be coming. There may be other abnormalities in his blood work, too, including abnormal sodium and potassium levels. You are in shock by the news because your dad has never had a kidney problem that you were aware of.

So what happened? His kidneys were "stunned" by the illness, dehydration, and the negative effect of the medications on his kidneys in this situation. When the body is physically stressed, the kidneys have built-in defense mechanisms to try to maintain normal kidney function. Depending on how badly the kidneys will be affected by an illness or other body stressors depends on one of three factors:

- *The severity of the illness.* The kidneys are in harmony with the rest of the body and will be affected by a severe illness. It is common to see the kidney function affected by a bad illness, especially in people who are admitted to the hospital.

- *The degree of kidney disease present.* Often, doctors will find that there was some degree of CKD present that no one ever knew about. The less kidney "reserve" one has, the less able the kidneys are to fully recover from significant body stressors like an acute illness.

- *The medications that interfere with the kidneys' built-in defense mechanisms.* Some medications get in the way of the kidneys' defense mechanisms as they try to maintain normal function in the face of a bad illness.

Let's review the effects of some of the medications that interfere with the kidneys.

ACE Inhibitors/ARBs

These classes of medication are effective in treating heart and kidney disease over a long-term basis. In this acute situation, however, when the body is not in its normal state, relaxing the kidney can actually make the kidney function worse. If your doctor is going to put you on one of these medications, understand that if you have an acute illness, nausea, vomiting, or diarrhea, you should not take it until those symptoms resolve. Your doctor will likely check your blood work to closely monitor your kidney function.

Diuretics

Many older patients may have a history of congestive heart failure or have significant problems with edema. From personal experience, I can tell you that many of them are deathly afraid of stopping their diuretic for fear of fluid building up in their lungs or legs, and the necessity of possibly having to go into the hospital. Yet when they have nausea, vomiting, and diarrhea, and are eating and drinking less, they can make themselves really dehydrated if they continue to take their diuretic. This can dramatically worsen their kidney function.

NSAIDS

Like diuretics and ACE inhibitors/ARBs, in a situation where the body is stressed, NSAIDS can stun the kidney and worsen kidney function. This is a different reaction than the nephritis or inflammatory response discussed in the prior section.

If your loved one complains to you of nausea, vomiting, or diarrhea, I strongly urge you to call his doctor and ask if any or all of the above medications should temporarily be stopped.

THE USE OF PHOSPHORUS-CONTAINING COMPOUNDS

Patients who are scheduled for colonoscopies are usually given oral phosphate-containing solutions as part of the preparation in order to cause a significant bowel movement before the procedure. However, there have been reports of such compounds causing acute kidney failure; in some cases the kidney function didn't return to normal. The term for this form of kidney failure is *acute phosphate nephropathy*. The combination of the patients being dehydrated from the preparatory agent in addition to the use of ACE inhibitors/ARBs and a diuretic is felt to be a contributing factor.

If you need to get a colonoscopy, question your doctor as to the type of preparation he is using. I would recommend avoiding the use of any phosphorus-containing enemas as they can affect kidney function. If you are on an ACE inhibitor/ARB or diuretic, ask which medications should be temporarily stopped prior to the procedure.

THE USE OF CONTRAST DYE OR GADOLINIUM IN IMAGING AND OTHER INTERVENTIONS

There are imaging studies such as CAT scans and MRIs that your doctor may ask you to obtain. In order to get a more detailed "picture" of what the doctor is looking for, you may be asked to get these studies using either contrast dye or a type of contrast called *gadolinium (gadolin-eum)*. If you have CKD, there are possible risks to the kidneys.

Contrast Dye for a CAT Scan

Your doctor may ask you to obtain a special kind of imaging study called a CAT scan. This can be of your head, chest, or abdomen—or a combination of all three depending on what he is looking for. You may be asked to obtain this study with intravenous contrast, which is a type of dye that is injected into a vein at the time of the study.

Depending on your level of kidney function, the use of such a dye can pose a risk to your kidneys. The higher the dose and concentration of the contrast used, the greater the risk. If you have CKD, there is a greater risk, as well. If you need to obtain a CAT scan, ask your doctor if dye needs to be used. When the answer is yes, there are a couple things you can do to minimize the risk to your kidneys. The first is to avoid using any diuretic or ACE inhibitor/ARB, at least on the day of the study. And the second is to increase your fluid intake at least by 25 to 50 percent the day before the study. The key is to talk with your doctor before any type of study like this is done.

Sometimes, on an emergent basis, you may not have the luxury of preparing beforehand. For example, some people come to the emergency room with severe shortness of breath, and the doctor may order a CAT scan with IV dye to make sure there is no clot in the lungs. As this is a life-threatening emergency, this type of study will be done as quickly as possible. Your doctor will be following your kidney function closely. And while the use of intravenous dye in imaging studies can affect kidney function, other, more invasive procedures can pose a greater risk.

Cardiac Catheterizations and Other Invasive Studies

With the degree of coronary artery disease (CAD) and peripheral vascular disease (PVD) in our society, procedures such as cardiac catheterizations and angiograms have saved both lives and limbs. We talked briefly about angiograms in Chapter 5 in the section concerning vascular disease and the kidney. These procedures have helped many patients open up clogged and diseased arteries, maintaining the blood flow of the heart and keeping their extremities intact. The above two procedures are referred to as *percutaneous (perk-yu-tane-eus)* interventions, as they access internal organs through a small puncture in the skin.

In these interventions, a cardiologist, vascular surgeon, or other trained doctor needs to look at the blood flow of the heart or extremity. To get an accurate assessment of the degree of blockage, it is necessary for the doctor to inject dye.

If a blockage is present in the artery, a specific type of intervention—an angioplasty (opening a narrowed vessel with a type of balloon)—may be performed. If needed, a stent, which is a device placed in the artery to keep the blood flow open, will be added. If this is the case, more dye may be needed to better see the affected area. As before, the more dye that is used the higher the risk of the kidney being affected. Other risks of this "dye nephropathy" include CKD, diabetes, and dehydration.

There are important precautions you can take to reduce these risks. Your doctor may suggest the following:

- You may be asked to come to the hospital one day before the procedure to get some intravenous fluids. Doing this keeps your kidneys "flushed" and is the best thing you can do to reduce the dye risk.

- Your doctor may ask you to take Mucomyst, an oral form of N-acetylcysteine (NAC), starting one day prior to the procedure. NAC is an herbal supplement with antioxidant activity. Taken twice a day for two days, it may have a protective effect on the kidney.

Between a Rock and a Hard Place

Procedures like cardiac catheterizations occur when people are in the hospital. A common scenario that doctors see is this:

A man comes into the hospital because of chest pain. He has both advanced CKD and bad heart disease. A cardiac catheterization is requested. In this scenario, both doctor and patient are between a rock and a hard place.

Without the cardiac catheterization, the man will likely continue to have heart problems. If the cardiac catheterization is performed, however, there is a risk of worsening kidney function, especially in the setting of advanced kidney disease. So what is the right answer to this situation?

The entire medical team will discuss all of the options with the patient. In the above scenario, without a cardiac intervention the heart will not get any better. Here, the man and his family elected to go ahead with the heart catheterization. He was given intravenous fluids and Mucormyst one day prior to the procedure. Fortunately, his kidney function remained stable.

In a situation like this, there are sometimes no right answers. In helping the heart, the kidneys can be affected. This is an example of why communication with the other members of the medical team and the patient is so important.

- If you are on the medication metformin (Glucophage) for diabetes, you will be asked to stop taking this medication for forty-eight hours prior to the procedure.

- Stop taking the ACE inhibitor/ARB at least twenty-four hours prior to the procedure.

As always, talk with your doctor about your options.

Magnetic Reasonance Imaging (MRI) and the Use of Gadolinium

In addition to CAT scans, MRIs are a common type of imaging procedure your doctor may order. Like CAT scans, they can be done with or without contrast. The type of contrast used in MRI studies, however, is called *gadolinium (gad-o-lin-eum)*. There have only been a few reports of MRI studies where gadolinium has been used and blamed as causing kidney failure. The more significant risk may be a skin condition called nephrogenic systemic fibrosis (NSF).

NSF was initially discovered several years ago when people would complain to their doctors about a bronzing or thickening of the skin. Biopsies of those areas revealed gadolinium in the layers of the skin. It was thought that the use of MRI, particularly in those with advanced kidney disease (GFR < 30 ml/min), increased the risk of this process. How this happens is still not quite known, and as of yet there is no recommended treatment.

If your doctor requests that you get an MRI, ask if the study is truly needed. If so, ask if gadolinium needs to be given. When it does, ask what will be done to minimize the potential toxicities of the suggested study. Depending on your kidney function, your doctor may suggest avoiding the use of gadolinium altogether (less than 30 percent) unless it is absolutely needed.

SUMMARY

It is important to understand the effects of the medications and imaging studies your doctor may prescribe for you. With every medication, every imaging study, and every procedure, it is important to assess the risks and benefits. *Will this medication benefit me? Could this imaging study or procedure hurt me or my kidneys in any way?* If you have kidney disease, and even if you don't, it is sometimes important enough to ask your doctor when not to take a medication as well as when to take one.

8

Complications of Chronic Kidney Disease and Standard Treatment Approaches

The complications caused by CKD impact our overall health and well-being. As CKD progresses, blood, bone, the pH (acid-base) balance, and heart health are affected. This chapter will familiarize you with these complications as well as their standard treatment approaches.

BLOOD HEALTH

As CKD progresses, the kidneys' ability to make the hormone *erythropoietin (erith-thro-po-eaten)* is greatly diminished. If you recall, the job of this hormone is to stimulate the bone marrow to make more red blood cells. When the number of red blood cells decreases, there is a decrease in the hemoglobin (Hgb) level. Remember that red blood cells contain Hgb, which carries oxygen to the body's cells. A low Hgb level can result in a condition called anemia. The normal ranges for Hgb are between 14 to15 mg/dl for men and 12 to 13 mg/dl for women, however an acceptable Hgb level for someone with CKD is between 11 to 12 mg/dl.

In addition to causing weakness and fatigue, anemia affects the heart. Since the body always tries to maintain balance, the heart will work harder to supply the body with much-needed oxygen. Over time, the overworked heart becomes worn down. Anemia is a contributing factor of heart disease and heart problems that can develop in CKD.

Treatment involves supplementing or replacing the erythropoietin that the kidneys no longer produce. One of the two following medications will be prescribed: epoetin alfa (Procrit) or darbepoetin alfa (Aranesp). Both are usually given by injection at the doctor's office. In certain circumstances, a patient or one of his family members can be trained to give these injections at home. The doctor, who is closely monitoring the Hgb levels, determines the dosage and injection schedule. The injection schedule can range from weekly to as far apart as every three to four weeks. Injections are usually withheld when an Hgb level is greater than 12. Note that the Hgb levels that doctors now use as guidelines may change in the future.

Procrit and Aranesp can raise the blood pressure; therefore, it is important that a blood pressure reading be done before injecting the medication. Your doctor will instruct you at what blood pressure to hold the medication; usually it is held when the systolic blood pressure is greater than 160, which is the top number on the blood pressure cuff. The technique for obtaining your blood pressure if you are doing injections at home is discussed in Part Three.

In order to get the maximum benefit from the injections, you need to have an adequate amount of iron stored in your body. If you are found to have low iron levels, a supplement can be prescribed. Sometimes iron levels are so low that your doctor may need to order an intravenous form of replacement.

It is important to note that a recent study has indicated a possible link between anemia replacement therapy and cancer progression in people already diagnosed with certain cancers. Nephrologists will collaborate with cancer doctors, or *oncologists (an-kala-gists)*, to provide optimal treatment and care.

BONE HEALTH

The overlapping and intersecting roles that calcium, phosphorus, vitamin D, and a hormone called the *parathyroid (para-thigh-roid)* hormone (or PTH for short) play keep bones healthy. A proper balance of each should always be maintained, because a rise in one can cause undesirable effects on the body. To prevent this complex relationship from going awry, the blood levels of calcium, phosphorus, PTH, and vitamin D are closely monitored.

One of the kidneys' functions is to get rid of the phosphorus in our diets. In CKD—usually Stage 3 and above—this is a difficult task for the kidneys to perform and the phosphorus levels can climb. A low-phosphorus diet is often an ideal treatment in theory, but very difficult to implement in practice. Phosphorus is a mineral found in most foods, and such a restricted diet is not usually tolerated by most people.

When blood work shows that your phosphorus levels are about 5.5 or higher, medications called phosphorus binders will more than likely be prescribed. They are taken with meals to prevent the body from absorbing the phosphorus consumed. These medications include calcium acetate (PhosLo), sevelamer acetate (Renvela), and lanthanum carbonate (Fosrenol). Dosage varies depending on your phosphorus levels and dietary intake.

If blood work shows that PTH levels are high, a kidney-specific type of vitamin D will be prescribed, called vitamin D analogues (ana-logs). If you recall from Chapter 2, another one of the kidneys' many functions is to transform some of the "normal" vitamin D in your body into a kidney-specific form. In the moderate to advanced stages of CKD, the kidneys can no longer do this properly. This kidney-specific vitamin D keeps the PTH levels in check. At moderate to severe kidney disease, your kidney doctor may likely prescribe a vitamin D analogue. These medications include calcitriol (Rocaltrol), paricalcitriol (Zemplar), and doxercalciferol (Hectorol). Again, the dosage will be adjusted depending on the corresponding calcium, phosphorus, and PTH levels.

ACID-BASE HEALTH

The body is constantly challenged to maintain a proper acid-base balance. An increased acidic state causes a condition called acidosis. Many factors can cause acid buildup, but diet—especially eating animal protein—and worsening kidney function are often the main culprits. The kidneys will again step up to the plate and work even harder to try to rid the body of the acid overload. However, diabetes and advanced kidney disease greatly reduce the kidneys' ability to flush the body of this excess acid.

Acidosis is not good for the cellular health of the body. As the imbalance increases, it can cause significant problems to the kidneys, the heart, and the bones. Acidosis can also increase the level of inflammation in the body and the kidneys.

If you remember the pool metaphor from Chapter 1, balancing the pH of the pool water requires adjusting the levels of the acid or base of the water. If there is too much acid in the blood, which is a common occurrence in advanced kidney disease, your doctor will prescribe a type of base, or baking-soda-like product called sodium bicarbonate. This can involve taking several pills; therefore, I try to use sodium citrate, which is a liquid form. Both bicarbonate and citrate can cause stomach upset and heartburn in certain individuals. Notify your doctor if you have any of these symptoms.

Your doctor will monitor your bicarbonate level on your blood work before any type of bicarbonate replacement is started. If approved for use, this medication will attempt to help neutralize the acid. Diet and other natural forms of bicarbonate replacement can also may help help reduce acid levels. There will be more discussion on this in Part Three.

HEART HEALTH

Progressive CKD significantly increases the risk of heart disease and heart-related deaths—just as heart disease can trigger damage to the kidneys. Hypertension, diabetes, high cholesterol, and high levels of inflammation are major components for both CKD and heart disease.

The treatment focuses on keeping all of the contributing factors in check, including maintaining adequate hemoglobin levels to prevent anemia; lowering bad cholesterol and triglyceride levels and raising good cholesterol levels; stabilizing blood pressure to maintain a level at least less than 130/80; monitoring salt intake; reducing urine protein (albumin) levels; reducing the cause and level of inflammation; and making dietary and lifestyle changes.

SUMMARY

The many health issues in kidney disease are complex, and that is why prevention and early detection are so important. The more advanced the kidney disease, the more the body is affected. Paying attention to the risk factors is very important; here, an ounce of prevention is worth far more than a pound of cure.

PART THREE

Complementary Treatment Approaches and Lifestyle Changes

Despite all of the incredible advances in medicine, we remain an unhealthy society. One out of every three Americans is obese and diabetes is affecting both teenagers and young people in record proportions. Moreover, there are perhaps thousands, if not millions of people walking around with undiagnosed kidney disease. Obesity, high blood pressure, diabetes, and kidney disease are all conditions that you can do something about. It is the simple things that matter the most—exercise, dietary changes, understanding the environment around you, and making the right life choices.

So what does this mean for you, the reader? It means that after you read Part Three you need to get moving. I mean this literally. You have to move, exercise, walk, swim, do some type of purposeful movement every day. In Chapter 9, the focus is on lifestyle changes everyone can do. This includes exercise, smoking cessation, stress reduction, and many other alterations to consider. We will also talk about the importance of getting a good night's sleep, and the effect that sleep apnea—one of the most under diagnosed conditions in this country—has on high blood pressure and kidney health.

Chapter 10 discusses how to make the right dietary choices. There is a specific "food education" that you will learn concerning kidney disease. Included in this detailed chapter is information on sodium restriction, potassium, and many other facets of kidney disease nutrition, with an emphasis on a more natural, vegetable-based diet. Examples for breakfast, lunch, and dinner are provided.

Chapter 11 focuses on vitamins and nutritional supplements. You will read about the many benefits that various vitamins and supplements can have when taken under the watchful eye of a doctor. Chapter 12 deals with herbal preparations and complementary medicines as they pertain to kidney disease. In kidney disease, you need to be very aware of the ingredients in the supplements that you take, because many contain potassium or have diuretic properties that can affect kidney function, especially if you have advanced kidney disease. Information on kidney cleansing and probiotics is also included.

Finally, Chapter 13 focuses on the intangibles that not only affect kidney health, but also make us whole human beings. Topics such as family support and the role of prayer are discussed. It's time to get started on the path toward a healthier you.

9

$\mathscr{L}$ifestyle Changes Everyone Can Make

This book has touched on many important issues concerning kidney disease. Yet this part of the book—this chapter in particular—is one of the most important. Why? Because *by changing your lifestyle, you can change your life.* By doing some of the things listed in this chapter, not only are you going to improve your kidney health, but you are also going to improve your overall health. Before undergoing any major lifestyle changes, first talk with your doctor and other health care providers. Keep in mind the changes listed below should only be used as general guidelines, as your situation may be different.

EXERCISING AND LOSING WEIGHT

We were put on this earth to move; our bodies were built for motion, not for remaining sedentary. There are many exercise books out there with all sorts of unique regimens. There are also many types of exercise machines, from stair climbers to rowing machines to abdominal machines promising to give you that six-pack look. All of this equipment is great, but the key is simply to find some way to move every day.

At the heart of all good exercise programs is *purposeful movement.* Walking every day for at least twenty to thirty minutes will benefit you. For optimal bone and muscle health, I advocate muscle training with light weights in addition to some type of aerobic exercise. If this is impossible, then just do whatever kind of purposeful movement you can each day.

With movement and proper dietary changes—to be discussed in Chapter 10—comes weight loss. If you recall, we talked about obesity and the harmful effect that excess weight has on kidney function. Even a weight loss of five to ten pounds can make a big difference, not only in lowering blood pressure but also in helping your kidney function. That's five or ten pounds your body no longer has to carry around, and less work for your kidneys, as well.

But what if you have trouble walking or can't walk at all? Many older patients have debilitating arthritis especially in their knees. If they are also overweight, walking around can be extremely difficult. If you fall into this category, here are some other options that can get your body moving with less strain:

- *Stationary Bike.* This is an excellent, minimal-impact exercise with great aerobic benefits. The bicycle is commonly used by rehabilitation specialists and physical therapists in most centers. You should start slow and gradually work up with each session. If you are able to use a regular bicycle, the fresh air and vitamin D you will obtain from the sun provides an added benefit. One reason many people stop using the stationary bike indoors is because they get bored. Listen to some music or work out with someone else while you exercise to help alleviate the boredom.

- *Swimming or Aqua Therapy.* Swimming is one of the best exercises you can do, as it works the entire body. Aqua therapy refers to specialized programs you can do in the water that focus on different parts of the body. Examples of this include walking or running in the water. You get the benefits of water resistance and your body doesn't receive the pounding it would have if you were running on land. I have had older patients in my practice who have benefited greatly from aqua therapy. You should first be evaluated by a licensed therapist or trainer to have the exercise program tailored to your individual needs.

- *Weight Training.* This should complement any type of aerobic exercise. As we get older, the building of muscle can not only help us burn calories more efficiently, it can also maintain and even improve our bone health. This is especially important in kidney disease. With weightlifting, the goal is not to get buff, but to get *toned*. Higher repetitions and lower poundage will improve strength and endurance. Before proceeding with any lifting program, you should obtain clearance from your doctor and your weightlifting program should be supervised by a qualified professional.

Any exercise program, even a walking program, can be difficult when you are just starting out. Begin slowly, and gradually build up the intensity each day. If your lifestyle has been fairly sedentary, consult with a qualified professional before starting your training regimen.

SMOKING CESSATION

In addition to the cancer risk—not just lung cancer, but also kidney and bladder cancer—and the effects of cigarette smoke on raising blood pressure, there is a direct toxic effect of smoking on kidney function. It is bad on the blood vessels because it accelerates the risk of atherosclerosis, and it also triggers an inflammatory reaction in the kidneys. Stopping smoking can directly improve your kidney health.

REDUCING EVERYDAY STRESSES IN YOUR LIFE

Everything in the body is interconnected. Up to this point we have only been talking about "body stressors" of the kidneys, including diabetes and hypertension. However, stress in its many forms, including psychological stress, affects our kidney health. Our lifestyles are full of stress; between monetary, economic, family, and work stress, we are constantly being bombarded by it. Most of us have no way of relieving this stress either, and the buildup of tension is not good. One of the added benefits of exercise, in addition to weight loss, is that it can be a great stress reliever. An important aspect of this is taking some "me time" each day; and meditation, yoga, and tai chi are all great ways to fit some in at home, without any special equipment.

Meditation

Everyone should set aside some quiet time each day, even if it is only for a few minutes. Through meditation, we are able to get centered and, for a few minutes each day, be free from the stresses that plague us. Meditation can take many forms and is different for everyone, but people who do some form of meditation have lower blood pressure, less heart problems, and better overall health. I highly recommend meditating on a daily basis.

Yoga

More than just a form of meditation, yoga is a great form of exercise. It increases total body flexibility and allows you to get centered. Speak with your doctor before embarking on such a program.

Tai Chi

This ancient Chinese exercise emphasizes purposeful but relaxed flowing movements. It is an excellent form of exercise and a great stress reliever. It also has been demonstrated to lower blood pressure, improve flexibility, and relieve chronic pain. Tai chi can be performed by anyone of any age.

GETTING A GOOD NIGHT'S SLEEP

Sleep is how our bodies restore themselves. Yet, even though it is so important, our society is very sleep deprived. At the very least, you should be getting eight hours each night. Any less than that can contribute to increased overall irritability and increased stress. While the quantity of sleep that you get is important, it is the *quality* of that sleep that is equally, if not more important.

When we are sleeping, there are changes occurring in our bodies. We are in a state of deep relaxation and regeneration. Our blood pressure should be at the lowest point of the day and our sleep should be restorative; we should wake up feeling refreshed.

For those with sleep apnea, however, their sleep is anything but restorative. It is interrupted; they may have periods where they stop breathing—apneas—or mini-periods where their breathing pattern is interrupted for less then a second. People with sleep apnea are often obese and they may have high blood pressure and kidney problems, as well. Sleep apnea is probably one of the most under diagnosed conditions in our country and is a common cause of high blood pressure that may be difficult to control.

If you have sleep apnea, your body may not be getting the necessary oxygen it needs at night. When that happens, your heart works harder, your blood pressure goes up, your quality of sleep suffers, and I believe the kidneys are also forced to work harder.

The worse the degree of sleep apnea, the worse the symptoms the sufferer will experience. At its extreme, people who have sleep apnea and their significant others will complain of nonstop snoring, and occasionally, of stopped breathing. Sufferers will wake up in the morning feeling very tired and can fall asleep at the drop of a dime anytime during the day. This is especially dangerous if the person has a long drive to work in the mornings or operates heavy machinery. For many people, the symptoms are not as dramatic. In my practice I recommend that anyone with high blood pressure that is resistant to treatment be evaluated for sleep apnea, even if they are not obese.

If your doctor suspects that you have sleep apnea, you will be asked to undergo a test called a *polysomnography (poly-sam- na-grafie)*, or sleep study. This type of testing occurs at a dedicated center called a sleep lab. The test is usually performed overnight, when the pattern of your sleeping can be closely monitored to determine if you have sleep apnea.

If you are diagnosed, there are a few different treatment options, the first of which is weight loss. Shedding some excess pounds can dramatically improve the quality of your sleep and reduce the degree of the sleep apnea. Second, you may be asked to refrain from alcohol, as this can worsen the apneic symptoms. Third, you may be asked to get fitted for a type of oxygen mask called a continuous positive airway pressure (CPAP) that provides necessary oxygen while you sleep. For some, these masks are cumbersome and can disrupt sleep even more, though. Another option, if you have either a large *uvula* *(you-view-la)*—the punching bag type thing in the back of your mouth—or large tonsils, is to see a doctor who specializes in disorders of the ears, nose, and throat. He may decide to remove them as they may be obstructing your breathing.

The take-home message is this: *Getting diagnosed and treated can save your life, likely help your blood pressure, and help both your kidney and overall health.*

MONITORING YOUR BLOOD PRESSURE AT HOME

With regards to the discussion concerning sleep apnea and its effect on blood pressure, it is important to note that you should be monitoring your blood pressure at home. Many people rely only on measurements obtained at doctors' offices or at the "automated blood pressure sites" found in most pharmacies and supermarkets. The problem with those options is that the results may not reflect your true blood pressure. Many people have "white-coat" hypertension when they go to a doctor's office, meaning that their blood pressure is high in the office, but normal at home or other places. Therefore, it is very important to monitor your own blood pressure at home to get a better idea of what it truly is.

MONITORING YOUR BLOOD SUGARS AT HOME

As with blood pressure, if you have been diagnosed with diabetes it is important to check your blood sugars at home. It is important to measure them before you eat, as well as after certain meals—termed *post-prandial (pran-d-e-al)* glucose. Having high blood sugars increases the workload and stress on the kidneys. It is surprising how many people do not check them at home, but rely solely on

Taking Your Blood Pressure at Home

When—notice I didn't say if—you start taking your blood pressure at home, it is important to pay attention to the following principles:

- *Position.* You should be sitting at a table, feet flat on the floor, with your arm extended and resting comfortably on the table. Your arm should be at about heart level. Wear a short-sleeved shirt or have your sleeves rolled up if you are not. The blood pressure reading should never be taken on top of clothing. Additionally, the blood pressure you take at home should be a *resting* blood pressure; you should be sitting for about five minutes before taking the reading.

- *Type of Cuff.* There are several different types of cuffs. One is the "standardized" manual blood pressure cuff, which is placed on the upper part of your arm and is similar to how the doctor takes your blood pressure at the office. This requires practice if you are going to do it yourself, unless you're going to have someone take it for you. Another is the digital cuff , which is an electronic device that will give a digital-type of readout along with the heart rate on the monitor.

- *Size of Cuff.* The cuff should wrap tightly around the arm with a little bit left over. For adults, there is an adult-size cuff and a large-size cuff. The size is very important. If the cuff is too small, the reading could be falsely elevated; if the cuff is too large, it will falsely give a lower reading. You should review the type and size of the cuff you are using with your doctor.

  Follow the directions for inflating the cuff if you are using a digital cuff. Record your blood pressure and bring your results as well as the cuff into the office. Your doctor may want to use your cuff and compare a blood pressure reading taken in his office to your at-home results to get a better idea of its accuracy. The take home point is to, no matter what, *take your blood pressure at home!*

measurements obtained at their doctor's office. You should discuss monitoring your blood sugars at home with your doctor, if you are not doing so already.

UNDERSTANDING WHICH
OVER-THE-COUNTER MEDICATIONS TO AVOID

In Chapter 6, we talked about commonly prescribed medications and their potentially adverse effects on kidney function. In this section, I would like to focus on common over-the-counter medications and their potential effects on kidney function.

Acetaminophen

Acetaminophen is a very commonly prescribed over-the-counter medication that is used for the treatment of mild pain, from everything to headaches to joints. Many people are aware of its detrimental effects on the liver, but it is important to remember that over time, it may have an effect on kidney function as well. This is not talked about much, but it usually refers to an effect of taking acetaminophen over years. There are no official recommendations regarding acetaminophen and kidney function, other than, of course, to use as little as possible.

Over-the-Counter NSAIDS

Used for the treatment of chronic pain, this category involves the use of common over-the-counter brands such as Motrin, Ibuprofen, Advil, and Aleve. We reviewed the mechanisms by which NSAIDS can affect kidney function in Chapter 7. The same pretty much holds true for all its varieties.

Yet again, this category puts patients and doctors between a rock and a hard place. There are many patients, specifically elderly patients, who are suffering from the debilitating effects of osteoarthritis of the back, hips, or knees. Without the use of the above-mentioned medications, they are still in pain. As doctors, we want to make sure we adequately treat the pain, yet want to restrict the amount of NSAID and Tylenol use as much as can be tolerated. It is a difficult quandary for both doctor and patient, without an easy answer. There are many natural alternatives, but again, talk with your doctor before trying any new medications or supplements.

Pseudoephedrine (Sudafed)

Many over-the-counter cold remedies may contain some degree of pseudoephedrine. If you have blood pressure problems, you should avoid taking anything with Sudafed in it if at all possible.

Weight Loss Supplements

There are many weight loss supplements on the grocery shelves these days. Commercials on television have popularized many of these products, especially to younger folks. While weight loss is important, it's how you go about losing the weight that matters. The goal is to lose it *safely and slowly.* There are ingredients in many of these supplements, such as natural energy boosters, that can not only raise blood pressure, but can have detrimental effects on kidney function. Before starting any weight loss supplement, talk with your doctor.

Body-building Products

If you have kidney disease, you need to watch products that contain excess protein and creatine, which is a supplement used to help athletes build muscle. Taking either or both of these supplements forces the kidneys to work harder. In the setting of strenuous exercise and dehydration, these supplements have the potential to cause some serious kidney damage. I would strongly advise against using these products in the setting of kidney disease; if you feel that you must, I would work closely with your doctor and avoid dehydration with exercise when taking these supplements.

Caffeinated Beverages

Caffeine can raise blood pressure and is detrimental to overall body health. You need to be aware of the amount of caffeine in drinks—especially energy drinks—if at all possible. Moreover, in addition to their caffeine content, many soft drinks including diet sodas contain an artificial sweetener called aspartame. Contrary to popular belief, some recent evidence demonstrates that aspartame may actually promote weight gain, not weight loss. In addition, the phosphoric acid in many types of cola is very bad for your bones. The high phosphorus content in soft drinks is not good if you have CKD.

UNDERSTANDING THE ENVIRONMENT AROUND YOU

It is very important to be aware of the environment and all of the things in it that can affect not only your kidney health, but also your overall health. Everything from the water we drink to the things we may be exposed to at home, in our yards, or at work, can affect our kidney function.

The Contents of Our Drinking Water

Having good, safe drinking water is vital to our health and well-being. If you were to examine the contents of your tap water, you would probably be surprised at the number of impurities you'd find. Examples of contaminants that could be in the water include metals such as cadmium, lead, and arsenic. Exposure to low levels of cadmium and lead over time is a significant risk factor for the development of CKD. Water can also be contaminated with high levels of bacteria. There may be increased risks of hypertension, kidney disease, and even hypertension during pregnancy after being exposed to bacteria-contaminated water. Other contaminants, such as forms of benzene and other chemicals and pesticides also exist in some tap waters, and can affect kidney function.

In addition to contaminants, a published report from the Associated Press in March 2008 demonstrated very minute amounts of many different medications in our water. These drugs have already affected fish and other marine life, but the long-term effects in humans are still unknown. It can't be good, though, either for your overall health or your kidney health.

You should find out about the drinking water contaminants as well as the safety level of the water in your state or local area. If you have well water, you should have it tested on a regular basis (visit www.epa.gov/safewater/dwinfo.htm). If you are using tap water, you should consider obtaining a water filter that will remove the impurities. In general, filtration is a method where the water is put through a material that removes the impurities, leaving you with a purer form of water.

There are many types of filtration systems out there, however two of the most common include distillation and reverse osmosis. Regarding distillation, water is heated until it boils and forms steam; this steam is then collected and stored. Reverse osmosis filters use a type of pressure to "push" water through a medium, resulting in a pure product. Ask your doctor or other health provider regarding which type of filter system would work for you.

A possible concern about filtration systems in general is that they can only "filter" down to a certain size. It is not clear if any water system can clear the very small materials like the trace amounts of medication described above. Though they can be costly, I do think that a good water filtration system can decrease the exposure risk. There is more information regarding different filtration systems in the Resources section at the end of the book (page 161).

Exposures at Work

With regards to kidney health, exposures to certain heavy metals, such as lead, mercury, and cadmium can affect your kidney function over time. Painters, those working on old houses, machinists, and the like should be aware of the environment in which they work for exposures that affect their kidney health.

KEEPING HYDRATED

Once you have established that your drinking water is safe, it is important to stay hydrated. Our bodies are 60 percent water, and keeping ourselves hydrated is important not only in keeping our systems healthy, but also in keeping our systems flushed.

How much you can drink depends on your overall situation. For someone with CKD, this is a loaded question. Some people in advanced stages of CKD may be restricted by how much they take in. Examples of such restrictions commonly prescribed by doctors include one liter (one liter is about one quart) or one and a half liters total for the whole day. If you also have a heart problem such as congestive heart failure (CHF) or significant problems with edema, your doctor may also place a restriction on how much you can drink on a daily basis. Please understand that fluid restriction means the *total* amount of fluid; this not only includes water, but tea, juice, and other beverages, as well.

Additionally, you may be asked to weigh yourself daily. If there are significant weight changes on a daily basis—either too much weight or too little weight—the amount of fluid you take in each day can change. *Weight that changes daily is reflective of water weight; weight that changes over longer periods of time is more reflective of changes in food intake.*

If your doctor has not placed a restriction on the amount of liquid you can take in, an acceptable approach is to drink when you are thirsty. You can also take in water through other sources, including food. This will be discussed further in the next chapter concerning diet.

SUMMARY

Our water, our environment, and even some of our over-the-counter medications can have toxic effects on our kidneys and overall health. Not only as consumers, but as people with CKD, we need to know what we are being exposed to, and what we can do to avoid it. Keep vigilant, and look closely at what you are putting in your mouth, because your kidneys could be affected.

10

$\mathcal{T}$he Importance of Eating Right

Eating right is something that all of us can and should do. This is especially true in kidney disease. *Food is power.* Consuming a well-balanced diet can help our bodies maintain good health and slow down—even improve—the progression of kidney disease.

This chapter discusses the complex dietary issues that many with CKD face. Before going any further, however, it is important to clarify the term "diet." A diet is not an abstinence regimen to lose weight; rather, it is a balanced way of eating and living. If you are overweight, weight loss is important. The key is losing it while still providing your body with the nutrition it needs. Many of us eat to excess and yet we are sufficiently lacking the nutrients our bodies require. You can eat less and still feel more satisfied by eating healthy. If you are tempted to eat sweets and empty-calorie junk foods when they are in your pantry, simply don't put those items in your grocery shopping cart. Your wallet, your waistline, and your health will all thank you.

A "kidney diet" can vary from person to person according to other medical conditions and the results of blood work. Deciding what to eat often becomes a juggling act, especially if diabetes—the leading cause of CKD—and hypertension—the second leading cause of CKD—are present. Depending on your stage of CKD, further food restrictions may be required.

In the first part of this chapter, we will be discussing general food guidelines in the setting of CKD, emphasizing natural rather than processed foods. You will gain an understanding of how nutritious food translates to decreased inflammation and body balance maintenance. You will also begin to understand how to make better food choices while still adhering to the many "dietary restrictions" you face. Always consult with your doctor and dietitian before attempting any dietary changes. This is important, especially if your kidney disease has progressed to stages four and five.

What is discussed in this chapter should concern only those with CKD who are not on dialysis, as CKD patients who are on dialysis have significantly different nutritional requirments.

LOWERING YOUR SODIUM INTAKE

One of the first conversations you had with your doctor likely included a discussion on sodium, with the recommendation to lower your sodium intake and omit the use of the salt shaker. The reason for this is that diseased kidneys cannot deal with the increased sodium of the present-day diet. A high sodium intake increases the risk of high blood pressure, edema, and in some cases, leads to congestive heart failure.

The Difference Between Sodium and Salt

Sodium chloride, or table salt, contains about 40 percent sodium. In general, a teaspoon of salt contains about 800 ml of sodium. With CKD, you should not add salt to your cooking or to your food at the table. You should also limit naturally salty foods. If your doctor has prescribed a fluid restriction, salt will increase your thirst, which can make it difficult to comply with her orders.

An additional, hidden source of sodium is found in over-the-counter medications. These include pain relievers, cough medicines, laxatives, effervescent tablets, and antacids. Research on pain relievers suggests that a high number of tablets and frequency of use can result in increased risks of high blood pressure in both men and women. Always consult with your doctor before taking any over-the-counter medications.

More on Fluid Restriction

In addition to restricting sodium, depending on your stage of kidney disease and other health issues, you may also be asked to watch the amount of fluids you take in. In the last chapter, we talked a little about the reasons for restricting fluid intake. Here we will talk about how to go about it. A prescribed fluid restriction includes all fluids, including fluids taken with medications, alcohol, coffee, cream, fruit, milk, popsicles, pudding, sauces, soft drinks, soda, and yogurt, including frozen yogurt. Ice cream, ice milk, and ice cubes are also considered. One ice cube equals 10 mls of liquid.

Some people find it easier to visually monitor their intake throughout the day by measuring out their total fluid allowance into a pitcher or other container every morning. This helps them ration their allowances throughout the day. After taking a drink, an equal amount of fluid is removed from the container. When the container is empty, the allotted fluid has been reached for the day.

Remember that any food that is liquid at room temperature also needs to be included as fluid intake. Don't forget those juicy fruits such as melons and citrus fruits, and also vegetables like cucumbers. Save up your allowance if you have a scheduled social event or will be celebrating a holiday in the evening.

Helpful Measurements to Remember:

Amount	Standard	Metric
1 tsp	1/4 oz	5 mls
1 tbsp	1/2 oz	15 mls
1/4 cup	2 oz	56 mls
1/2 cup	4 oz	110 mls
1 cup	8 oz	25 mls
	1 oz	28 to 30 g

Examples of Foods High in Sodium

Many foods contain traces of sodium, but processed foods can contain very high amounts. Most people already know that snacks such as chips, crackers, pretzels, etc, are packed with sodium. However, they are typically unaware of unexpected sources of sodium such as canned foods, processed meats and cheeses, ready-made meals, gravy mixes and sauces, stuffing, bouillon cubes, and other processed foods. This is why it is so important to read food labels and find out the amount of sodium each item has. To give you an example, certain types of canned soups can have as much as 1 g (1000 mg) of sodium in one can. If you are on a sodium restriction, then by consuming that soup you will have already met more than half of your total daily requirement.

Sodium Allowance

In general, you should restrict your sodium intake to no more than 2 g (or 2000 mg) daily. If you have advanced CKD, significant edema, or congestive heart failure, then your doctor may discuss lowering it even further, to about 1500 mg daily. This amount is not set in stone and can vary if your health condition changes. For example, if you were to get a "stomach bug" and experience some diarrhea, your doctor may instruct you to eat more sodium-rich foods to replace what you are losing. In the case of diarrhea, for example, you may also be asked to drink more fluids in order to prevent dehydration. It's important to communicate with your doctor if you notice any changes in health.

WATCHING YOUR POTASSIUM INTAKE

Declining kidney function and some prescribed medications can alter potassium levels. Routine blood tests will determine if potassium needs to be increased or restricted. Some people with CKD may need to curb their intake of food and beverages that are high in potassium, because in diabetes or advanced CKD—stages four or five—the kidneys can have trouble getting rid of the extra potassium.

High potassium levels in the blood can also affect heart function. Think of the heart as a big electrical circuit; if the potassium levels get too high, it can short circuit the heart and even lead to life-threatening arrhythmias—abnormal electrical rhythms of the heart. If your potassium levels tend to be high, your doctor will be monitoring you closely with blood work.

Normal Potassium Levels

As reported on your blood work report, a normal potassium level is between 3.5 and 5.0 milliequivalents (meq). Levels higher than 5.5 warrant close monitoring, more dietary restrictions of potassium, a change in medication, or active treatment for the potassium depend-

---

Potassium Restriction

Generally, severe potassium restricted diets allow for about 2000 mg of potassium daily. More modest restrictions are 3000 mg a day. The following are several examples of foods and their potassium contents:

High Potassium Foods (containing 225 to 500 mg per serving)

Fruits: Apricots, Avocados, Bananas, Dates, Nectarine, Oranges, Peaches, Prunes

Drinks: Vegetable, Orange, and Tomato Juice (4 oz)

Vegetables: Artichokes, Beans (kidney, lima, navy, pinto) and Greens (collard, mustard, turnip) (4 oz). Also included are all types of nuts (1 oz to a 1/2 cup depending on the nut), potatoes (4 oz or 1 small), spinach (4 oz), tomatoes, tomato sauce (4 oz), yams and sweet potatoes (4 oz)

Medium Potassium Foods (containing 150 to 225 mg per serving)

Fruits: Apple, fruit cocktail (4 oz), papaya, and pears

Drinks: Grapefruit and pineapple juice (4 oz)

Vegetables: Broccoli (4 oz), Brussels sprouts (4 oz), celery (4 oz), mushrooms (4 oz)

Low Potassium Foods (containing 150 mg per serving)

Fruits: Grapes (4oz), pineapple (4 oz), strawberries (4 oz), watermelon (4oz)

Drinks: Apple juice (4 oz), lemonade (8 oz)

Vegetables: Asparagus, cabbage (4 oz), cauliflower (4 oz), corn (4 oz), cucumber (4 oz), lettuce (4 oz), onions (4 oz), summer squash (4 oz)

ing on how high the level is. Your doctor will discuss the various treatment options with you.

Reading Food Labels

When grocery shopping, read the food labels. You should know the nutritional value of what you are buying. Many food labels display the sodium content but not the potassium content. *This, however, does not mean that those foods are without potassium or other electrolytes and minerals.* Rather, it means that you have to search for more information regarding the nutritional value. To do so, you can visit the website of that particular product, or you can visit excellent websites like www.fns.usda.gov or www.nutritiondata.com. A listing of other informative websites can be found in the Resources section (page 161).

LOWERING YOUR PROTEIN INTAKE

In the United States, most of us eat way more protein than we need. Having protein in the urine forces your kidneys to work harder, and in CKD they do not cope well with the accumulated protein overload. One of the mainstays of treatment is a diet lower in protein. If you have CKD, the general recommendation with regards to dietary protein is that you should take in no more than 0.6 to 0.8 g/kg of body weight daily. These calculations are again done using the metric system (just to make it more confusing!).

For calculations concerning body weight, the first step is to convert your body weight from pounds to kilograms. To do this, simply divide your weight in pounds by 2.2 to get your weight in kilograms (2.2 kg = 1 lb). For example, a body weight of 150 lbs, divided by 2.2, is equal to 68 kg of body weight. The amount of allowable protein, then, is 68 g x 0.8, which equals about 55 total g of protein daily.

There is a general misconception that protein can only be obtained from animal sources. Animals are good sources of protein, but they are often high in saturated fat and a main source of dietary cholesterol. Some plants, however, are equally good sources of protein and they have the added benefits of being low in saturated and high in fiber. One concern had been that by eliminating all animal

Is an Even Lower Protein Intake Better?

This has been a very controversial topic in nephrology. If a low-protein diet decreases the workload of the kidneys, wouldn't eating even lower amounts be even better? There have been major studies examining both views that have found very different results. In the mid-1990s, studies were done which demonstrated that eating very low-protein diets—in the range of 0.2 mg/kg a day—supplemented with amino acids, reduced the amount of protein in the urine. For those with very advanced kidney disease, it delayed the time until dialysis was started.

However, in a study published in 2009, patients who were on a moderately low-protein diet—0.5 to 0.6 g/kg of body weight—were compared to those on a very low-protein diet—0.2 g/kg of body weight. Both groups of patients were followed closely by their doctors for years. Those on a very low-protein diet did not fare any better than those on the higher-protein diet. It was also suggested by the study that those on a very low-protein diet may have a higher mortality. The one factor that made a significant difference in preventing kidney disease from worsening was maintaining a lower blood pressure.

Most nephrologists are recommending a moderately lower protein intake of 0.6 to 0.8 g/kg. It also may mean that there are factors other than the amount of protein that can contribute to a worsening of kidney disease. In addition to a higher blood pressure, I submit that this also includes a *sustained inflammatory response.*

sources of protein, you were not getting all of the different types of protein your body requires. By combining many plant sources, however, daily protein needs can be met.

In addition to plants, other non-animal sources of protein include soy, tofu (a soy-based food), and whole grains. If it is determined that you need additional protein in your diet, you can see that you have many supplemental sources to choose from, both soy- and vegetable-based. Always talk with your doctor before trying a new supplement.

A concern in restricting protein worth mentioning is the potential for malnutrition. Your doctor will order routine blood work to assess albumin and prealbumin levels. These tests measure the nutritional status in your body. High protein diets or body-building protein supplements are strictly off-limits unless otherwise directed by your doctor or dietitian.

RESTRICTING PHOSPHORUS IN THE DIET

Phosphorus is an important mineral found in all cells of the body. When joined with calcium, it helps maintain the integrity of our teeth and bones. As CKD progresses, the kidneys can no longer eliminate excess phosphorus to maintain body balance, and as a result, phosphorus accumulates in the blood.

When this happens, calcium is leached from the bones and can also build up in the blood, which can cause changes in bone health as well as heart and blood vessel damage. Blood work will again indicate if dietary changes or medication is needed. If results indicate that the phosphorus level is too high, the doctor will more than likely prescribe a medication called a phosphate binder.

Normal Phosphorus Levels

A normal phosphorus level, as reported in your blood work, is 2.5 to 4.5 meq. When the number reaches 5.5 or higher, your doctor may talk with you about using a phosphorus binder, as discussed in the earlier chapters.

Sources of Phosphorus

Phosphorus is found in most foods, but mainly in protein-based foods, such as meat, poultry, fish, and dairy. Therefore, restricting dietary protein will limit the amount of phosphorus consumed.

Phosphorus is also found in much smaller quantities in fruits and vegetables. You should be aware of hidden sources of phosphorus, as well. For example, phosphate additives are added to commercially prepared foods and soft drinks, especially colas. As with potassium, the phosphorus content may not be listed on all food labels. You need to be aware of the phosphorus content of the food that you buy. In general, the amount of phosphorus restricted is to about 700 to 1000 mg each day.

KEEPING AN EYE ON MAGNESIUM INTAKE

Magnesium is a mineral that is important in bone and nerve health. Normal levels as reported on blood work are approximately 1.6 to 2.0 mg. In the advanced stages of CKD, the kidneys can have trouble eliminating excess magnesium.

Pay attention to how much magnesium you are consuming. In addition to vegetables and whole grains, magnesium is also found in over-the-counter medications such as laxatives, milk of magnesia, epsom salts, many antacids, and pain relievers. Over-consumption of these products could put you at risk for magnesium toxicity. It is very important that your doctor know about all of the over-the-counter medications you are taking, including multivitamins containing potassium and magnesium. Again, blood work will dictate if restrictions are necessary.

UNDERSTANDING FOOD CHOICES

In our fast paced lives, quick and easy have become a priority. Convenience, however, has its consequences. When foods are processed they are changed from their natural states and many healthy nutrients are removed, resulting in foods that are high in saturated fats, transfats, sugar, salt, artificial ingredients, additives, and preservatives. If you have ever read the labeled ingredients of processed foods, I bet you have found that you can't pronounce most of them, let alone have any idea as to what they are. And don't let minimalistic labels fool you, either. Manufacturers are not required to list additives they consider safe, so their labels can read as little as "artificial color and flavor." In addition, the serving sizes of many prepared foods, such as certain frozen dinners, are much more than one person could possibly eat at a sitting

Whole foods, on the other hand, provide you with numerous natural benefits. The term whole foods includes vegetables, fruits, and grains, all of which are loaded with fiber, minerals, and vitamins. Studies indicate that whole grain foods significantly lower the risk of developing heart disease and strokes, and possibly diabetes and other chronic conditions.

When possible, buy organic fruits and vegetables in season. Organic refers to the way agricultural products are grown. To be organic, the crops must be grown in safe soil, have no modifications, and be kept separate from conventional products. Farmers are not allowed to use synthetic pesticides, bioengineered genes (GMOs), petroleum-based fertilizers, or sewage sludge-based fertilizers. You may find that organic fruits and vegetables spoil faster because they aren't treated with waxes or preservatives. If fresh is not available, frozen fruits and vegetables are acceptable.

Even with whole foods, it is important to check the labels with regards to potassium and phosphorus content. In advanced stages of CKD, more restrictions may be prescribed and you will have to be more selective in food choices.

When choosing any food or dietary plan, there are a few other things to keep in mind. First, as CKD is a state of inflammation, any diet considered should be anti-inflammatory in nature. A vegetarian-based diet is very helpful in this regard. Second, a kidney-based diet should reduce the body's acidity, because the build up of acid in the body affects kidney, bone, and total body health, and worsens inflammation. Foods that contribute to an acidosis, like meat protein, should be eliminated from the diet, and foods that can counter the acid effect on the body should be emphasized. Finally, remember that a vegetarian-based diet is kidney and total-body healthy. In many ways, this is a restating of point number one, but that's how important it is. Vegetables have potent anti-inflammatory properties, and those who are on vegetarian-based diets typically live longer and have a better quality of life.

A REVIEW OF SOME COMMON DIETS

We are now going to review some of the conditions from the prior chapters in the context of which dietary options are best for them.

Hypertension and the DASH Diet

One of the most well-studied diets that has been demonstrated to have a dramatic effect on lowering blood pressure and preserving kidney function is the Dietary Approaches to Stop Hypertension (DASH) diet plan. Endorsed by organizations like the American Heart Association, DASH has at its core an emphasis on reducing salt intake and eating fruits, vegetables, and low fat foods. A recent article demonstrated that following the DASH diet reduced the incidence of heart failure.

The DASH diet, with its emphasis on vegetables, also has an emphasis on high potassium intake. If you have stage one or stage two kidney disease, this diet is an excellent option because it has a significant anti-inflammatory effect. You may have to watch your choices with regards to high potassium fruits and vegetables, but this is usually not too much of a problem in early kidney disease. If you have advanced CKD or problems with high potassium, then you need to be more careful in your food choices and make a point to discuss your diet with your doctor.

There are great many recipes and options with this diet. Cookbooks exist that give step-by-step plans regarding how to best utilize DASH. See the Resources section for more information (page 161).

Diabetes and the Glycemic Index

If you have diabetes, one of the cornerstones of any eating plan is paying attention to the type and amount of carbohydrates you consume. Because of this, it is important to understand the glycemic index, which categorizes the effect that different carbohydrates can have on raising your blood sugar levels.

Eating carbohydrates that are lower on the glycemic index can increase your body's responsiveness to insulin. One of the hallmarks of this low-glycemic diet is again its emphasis on whole grains, fruits, and vegetables. As before, you will have to watch the type of vegetables and fruits that you eat with regards to their potassium content. This type of diet plan is tremendous and can dramatically improve control of your blood sugars.

That being said, it is important to remember that in kidney disease, insulin can stay in the blood longer than it normally should. This is true for the insulin that your body makes, as well as for the insulin that your doctor may be prescribing for you. With any change in diet—changing the amount and types of carbohydrates that you are eating, for example—you may also need to reduce the amount of insulin that you are taking. If you do not, you will increase your risk of running a low blood sugar. Watch this with other groups of "diabetic medications" that you may be on, as well. An example is a class of diabetes medications called *sulfonylureas (sole-fon-il-your-e-as)*. Your doctor may need to adjust them depending on your kidney function and blood sugar levels.

The Atkins Diet

The Atkins diet has at its essence a very high-protein, high-fat model with little or no carbohydrates allowed. By putting your body in a state of *ketosis (kee-toe-sis)*, or fatty acid breakdown, it can help with weight loss, blood sugar control, and cholesterol level lowering.

The downside is that the high protein load can be shocking to the kidneys. Forced to eliminate even more protein, the kidneys work harder, which may cause a worsening of kidney function. Therefore, I cannot endorse this diet in the setting of kidney disease.

The Acid-Alkaline Diet

The acid-alkaline diet works on the principle that our bodies, which are geared towards balance, need to be at a neutral pH level. Our blood pH—a measure of the level of the acidity or alkalinity in the blood—normally runs slightly basic; however, many of us who consume Western-based diets are guilty of eating more acid-forming foods, including animal protein, which result in high acid levels in the blood. When the acid levels in the blood rise, it is thought to be a major contributor to illness and other health problems, including a worsening of inflammation. As kidney disease worsens, there is a problem with acid buildup in the blood. In certain diseases like diabetes, people may be even more predisposed to states of acidosis even with mild kidney disease.

Many fruits and vegetables have more of an alkaline bent to maintain total body balance and decrease inflammation. But while they may be more alkaline, they also have a very moderate to high potassium content, and the amounts consumed need to be watched closely. Vegetables may be a better option. Broccoli, Brussels sprouts, beets, eggplant, green beans, cabbage, cucumber, lettuce, onions, radishes, summer squash, turnips, and water chestnuts have a low-to-moderate potassium content and are more alkaline. I recommend trying to include foods with an alkaline base, but careful attention needs to be paid to the potassium content of what you are eating. This requires a nutritional understanding of each piece of food you eat.

LIQUIDS AND ACIDOSIS

As stated before, advanced kidney disease reflects a state of acidosis, and as discussed in Chapter 8, medications like bicarbonate are prescribed to try to neutralize this acid effect. Often, however, this requires a lot of pills or citrate, a liquid form of the bicarbonate; and these medications are not tolerated well, as they can cause an upset stomach and heartburn.

Luckily, there are some tastier liquid alternatives that may help. Since many of you with CKD are restricted in how much you can drink, though, you need to be smart about it. And after all, shouldn't what you drink be as important as what you eat?

Alkalized Water

Many patients do not tolerate bicarbonate. For those who do, bicarbonate may not always be strong enough to counter the effects of acid buildup in the body. That is where alkalized water can help. Alkalized water is not only filtered, but with a pH of about 9 to 11, it has more of an alkaline pH than normal water, which is about 6.5 to 8.

There is water that is prepared already at this pH and there are ways of making it yourself. For instance, if you are using water that is filtered, the addition of pH drops can make the water more alkaline. Another option to increase the pH of filtered water is to add lemon or lime. A good guideline is one teaspoon of lemon or lime to one quart of water. Lemon is converted to citrate in the body, which helps neutralize the body's acidity. The amount of potassium in the lemon is very small, but be aware of the potassium content of alkalized water if you choose to buy it.

The Role of Juicing

Juicing is a great way to not only get the anti-inflammatory and antioxidant effects of fresh fruits and vegetables, but also to benefit from the alkaline effect of the fruits and vegetables you put in your drink. Again, it is important to watch the potassium content of the vegetables and fruits you choose.

A great juice drink my mother makes combines an apple (for flavor) with the three C's: cabbage, cucumbers, and carrots. You can vary what you put in the juice drink depending on your potassium restrictions. I would only recommend one fruit per drink, and in most cases, an apple, lemon, or lime should be the fruit added. Many other fruits are more acidic and can have a high glycemic index load, which you need to watch out for if you have diabetes.

Even on the most severe fluid restriction, juices can be enjoyed. For example, a 4 or 8 oz glass of freshly made juice in the morning is perfectly fine. For some, it can even take the place of the breakfast meal. Another option would be to have a 4 or 8 oz glass of alkaline water with a squeeze of fresh lemon or lime. This also provides a great start to the day. If you are not on a severe fluid restriction, you can choose to have a glass with dinner as well.

EXAMPLES OF DIETARY ALTERNATIVES

The best advice I can offer you is to be open and willing to change. For example, switching to a vegetable-based diet represents a radical change and is not easy for many; however, it can drastically improve your health. Moreover, most of us were raised to finish everything on our plates. Dinner was meat and potatoes, with maybe a soft drink or some other artificial drink to wash it down. Unhealthy eating behaviors were also instilled in many of us as teenagers, when fried food became our staple. Burgers and fries went hand in hand with zits and rock and roll.

Don't be afraid to kick those habits. The transition doesn't have to be difficult. Food can be tasty *and* nutritious. You just have to make the decision to change to a healthier lifestyle.

With each progressive stage of CKD, you should discuss dietary choices with your doctor and dietitian. Many of these dietary programs are individualized. A sampling of dietary options is presented below; but again, your particular situation may be somewhat different, so stay flexible.

Breakfast Examples

The following information represents options for changing your breakfast selections. The choices here reflect more natural and healthy alternatives to "traditional" breakfast foods.

Eggs

Instead of eating bacon and eggs for breakfast, consider trying an egg white vegetable omelet. Two large organic egg whites have approximately 110 mg of sodium, 110 to 120 mg of potassium, 10 mg of phosphorus, and 3.5 g of protein. Add 1/2 cup of raw, chopped broccoli (15 mg of sodium, 150 mg of potassium, 30 mg of phosphorus, and 1.3 g of protein), and 1/4 cup of chopped raw onion (6 mg of sodium, 55 mg of potassium, 11 mg of phosphorus, and 0.5 g of protein).

Mix and match your portion size and vegetable choice according to your dietary restrictions. The key is substituting the vegetables for bacon, and egg white for egg yolk. Other protein substitutes include tofu (a six-ounce portion of Mori-Nu soft, silken tofu provides 8 mg of sodium, 300 mg of potassium, 105 mg of phosphorus and 8 g of protein) and tempeh.

Cereal

Instead of high sugar breakfast cereals, consider trying a sprouted whole grain cereal. A brand that I recommend is Ezekiel. 1/2 cup of Ezekiel Golden Flax Organic Cereal provides 190 mg of sodium, 190 mg of potassium, 8 g of protein, and no sugar.

Instead of topping the cereal with cow's milk, consider using soy milk or rice milk. 1/2 cup of soy milk has approximately 15 mg of sodium, 170 mg of potassium, 60 mg of phosphorus, and 6.7 g of protein. Soy milk can have sugar, but there is an unsweetened option made by Organic Valley Farms.

Bread

Instead of a bagel, consider trying sprouted bread. One slice of Ezekiel Sesame Sprouted Grain Bread has only 80 mg of sodium, 75 mg of potassium, 4 g of protein, and no sugar. Additionally, it has only 8 percent of the total daily phosphorus requirements, which is low. Gluten-free sprouted bread is also if you have celiac disease.

Lunch Examples

For many of us, we are at work and only have an hour--if that--for lunch. We want something quick and light, yet nutritious. For the examples discussed below, you may choose to increase your portion size at lunch if it is your main meal day of the day. It is important to make dietary choices that work for your lifestyle and schedule.

Salad

Instead of salad as an appetizer, consider it as a main course. Raw vegetables are a good source of fiber and nutrition. Your salad should contain at least 1 cup of iceberg lettuce and 1 cup of romaine lettuce. 1 cup of romaine lettuce provides little sodium, 167 mg of potassium, 25 mg of phosphorus, and 1 g of protein. In contrast, 1 cup of iceberg lettuce has about a third less of sodium, and about 50 percent less phosphorus.

You can add almost anything to the lettuce. Consider carrots, either sliced or grated (a 7.5 inch carrot provides 50 mg of sodium, 230 mg of potassium, 25 mg of phosphorus, and a little less than 1 g of protein). Other options include cucumbers, peppers, spinach, and kale (1/2 cup of chopped raw kale provides 15 mg of sodium, 150 mg of potassium, 20 mg of phosphorus, and 2.2 g of protein). Top it off with oil and balsamic vinaigrette and you have a delicious lunch.

Sandwiches

Instead of a foot-long hoagie with fries for lunch, consider organic pita bread. A small 4-inch-diameter bread has anywhere from 60 to 120 mg of sodium, 50 mg of potassium, and 3 g of protein, with little or no sugar and fat. The phosphorus content is about 25 to 30 mg for this serving size. You can stuff the pita with any type of vegetable, as discussed in the case of the omelet, to make a vegetable sandwich.

Soup

Instead of a meaty cream-based soup, choose a broth-based vegetable soup instead. You can make any type of vegetable into a soup. Simply add vegetables of your choice to some vegetable broth and you are on your way.

Dinner Examples

Continuing this theme, reevaluate what you are eating for dinner. Perhaps you can make some healthier selections and discover a few tasty new foods.

Pasta

Instead of spaghetti, consider trying spaghetti winter squash. 1 cup boiled squash provides 28 mg of sodium, 181 mg of potassium, 22 mg of phosphorus, and 1 g of protein. Summer squash has an even lower amount of potassium.

If you can't give up actual pasta, at least consider whole wheat or whole grain varieties. 3/4 cup of whole wheat penne pasta from Heartland contains no sodium, no potassium, only 2 g of sugar, and 7 g of protein. Another option is quinoa (keen-wa). 1/2 cup of cooked quinoa contains only 7 mg of sodium, 140 mg of potassium, and 160 mg of phosphorus. It has a very low glycemic index score and provides 4 g protein.

Tacos and Burritos

Instead of corn tortillas, consider using a brown rice tortilla when making tacos and burritos. One wheat-free, gluten-free tortilla contains only 160 mg of sodium and 95 mg of potassium. It has no sugar, about 100 to 150 mg of phosphorus, and each provides 2 g of protein. Here again, you can add vegetables of your choice depending on your potassium requirements.

SPECIAL CIRCUMSTANCES

One of my reasons for espousing natural and healthy food choices in the face of kidney disease is that food can not only heal, it can also hurt. For those with certain forms of nephritis or the nephrotic syndrome, these words ring very true. The following information is useful in the face of special circumstances.

Glomerulonephritis (GN) and the Nephrotic Syndrome (NS)

In Chapter 6, we talked in depth about the role that food allergies may have in getting GN or NS. If you have been diagnosed with one of these syndromes, your diet should be as anti-inflammatory as possible in order to remove any possible exposure to contributing factors in foods. As you read, it can be very hard to pinpoint the exact allergy. Therefore, I would strongly recommend avoiding all dairy and processed food.

An interesting medical article suggested that celiac disease may be more common than once thought, and it is my opinion that it may be wise to consider a gluten-free diet.

Acidosis

If you have advanced CKD (stage four or five), or if your doctor says you have acidosis due to kidney disease or diabetes (this can happen here in the early stages), I would ask you to consider the use of alkalized water, plus the consumption of those vegetables that produce more alkalinity in the blood. Again, discuss all changes with your doctor before trying them. If you choose to use a pH booster, be sure you are aware of the potassium content.

SUMMARY

There are several important take-away points from this chapter, and I think they are most clear in list form. Now that you have completed this chapter, you should know a little about each of the following points:

• Blood tests are important in measuring sodium, potassium, magnesium, and protein levels.

• Dietary restrictions may be prescribed to preserve remaining kidney function

• If a fluid restriction is prescribed, you will need to keep track of fluid intake. This includes all foods that are liquid at room temperature, in addition to ice, ice cream, gelatin, gravies, sauces, and soups. Also, many fruits contain large amounts of water.

• Read nutrition labels and also be aware of hidden sources of salt, potassium, and phosphorus. If you have access to a computer, check nutrient database sites for additional information.

• Be vigilant with over the counter medications and make sure that your doctor is aware of all medications, herbal preparations, and vitamin and mineral supplements.

• Be knowledgeable about alternative food choices for optimal well-being and preservation of kidney function.

Food can have the power to change your health, but only you have the power to actually make it happen. In CKD, there are many things you have to pay attention to in terms of restrictions, but you don't have to do it alone. Remember, you have a plethora of resources at your disposal, as well as your doctor and dietitian to fall back on. Talk with your doctor and dietitian about creating an individualized diet plan, as everyone's needs are different.

11

$\mathscr{V}$itamins, Minerals, and Other Nutritional Supplements

In addition to changing your diet, there are other nutritional supplements that you may need to take depending on the cause and stage of CKD. Vitamins, minerals, and nutritional supplements in no way replace a good diet, but are important in maintaining nutrition and total body balance. In this chapter, we will discuss how vitamins and nutritional supplementation can be used in kidney disease.

THE OPTIMAL DOSAGE

In many cases, the dosage of a particular supplement may need to be changed because of kidney disease. The dose is often reduced, but in other instances the supplement may have more benefits at higher doses. For example, Thiamine, or Vitamin B1, may reduce proteinuria at a higher-than-normal dose. The "optimal dose" of many supplements still needs to be further studied. This chapter should only be used as a guide. Talk with your physician before making any changes in your current nutritional program.

THE VITAMINS

The following vitamins are generally safe in kidney disease; however, the dosage and frequency will depend on your stage of CKD,

Natural Versus Synthetic

Many types of vitamins and supplements are either natural or synthetic. The synthetic vitamins are harder for the body to break down and digest, whereas the more natural vitamins are easier on the stomach and better absorbed in the body. If possible, it pays to get the more natural form.

dietary regimen, and other medical problems. I try to have many of my patients on some combination of the vitamins listed below.

Vitamins

If you have been following a low-protein, vegetarian-based diet, you may need to take a vitamin B_{12} supplement, as it is commonly found in meat and animal products. On a vegetarian diet, you may be deficient in this vitamin. Low levels can contribute to nerve problems and anemia. As you will read below, B_{12} may also be important in maintaining bone health. If your doctor feels you may be deficient in this vitamin, she may order a blood test that can measure the level of B_{12} in the body.

Low levels of vitamin B_9, or folic acid, may play a role in the development of atherosclerosis. If you are on a vegetarian-based diet, you do not need folic acid supplementation, as B_9 is found in many leafy greens--though you may be taking a multivitamin, which will usually contain some amount of folic acid anyway. Vitamin B1, or thiamine, may help in reducing proteinuria. In one study, patients with type 2 diabetes and proteinuria were given thiamine at doses of 300 mg daily compared to a placebo group. After three months, the group taking the higher dose of thiamine experienced a decrease in the amount of proteinuria. This needs further research as the optimal dose and duration of therapy with thiamine is still unknown. However, this study suggests that higher doses of thiamine may lower the protein levels even more.

In a related study, it was suggested that the combination of high-dose thiamine and *benfotiamine (ben-fo-tya-mine)*—a manufactured form of thiamine—decreased the amount of proteinuria.

The B vitamins are important regulators of homocysteine (homo-sis-teen), an amino acid that is associated with heart disease at high blood levels, although this connection is still somewhat controversial. There may also be an association with elevated homocysteine levels and osteoporosis; although again, this needs more research. In one study, blood tests showing high homocysteine levels and low vitamin B_{12} levels were associated with an increased risk of bone fractures. Homocysteine levels can be elevated in CKD. More research is needed, but taking a B-complex vitamin daily seems reasonable pending further research into this area.

If no proteinuria is present, I would recommend taking one B-complex vitamin a day. If your vitamin B_{12} level as measured in the blood is low, you may need an additional daily B_{12} supplement. If you have diabetes and proteinuria, supplementing with thiamine at a dose of 200 or 300 mg a day (two to three tablets at 100 mg each) seems reasonable until more studies are done. If you have any type of cancer, talk to your doctor before either starting thiamine or increasing your thiamine dosage.

Vitamin C

Vitamin C is great for keeping the immune system healthy and is a known antioxidant. It also helps your body absorb iron better and more efficiently, so if you are taking an iron supplement orally, take vitamin C supplement at the same time.

In addition, a study suggests that vitamin C may play an important role in our bone health, as well as help in the treatment of anemia in CKD. A lab-based study proposes that high-dose vitamin C may have an antioxidant or protective effect on the kidneys, although a comparative study has not been done in humans.

Too high of a dose of vitamin C can affect the kidneys, as it can cause *oxalate (ox-ul-late)* to build up in the kidneys. Oxalate is a by-product of vitamin C; if too much vitamin C is eaten in the diet, the levels of oxalate can build up and be toxic to the kidneys. In addition, it can increase the risk of kidney stones.

As Vitamin C is abundant in fruits and vegetables, there is likely no need to take a vitamin C supplement if you are on a vegetarian diet. If you are taking an iron supplement, as many with anemia and CKD are, then I would take no more than a total of 125 to 250 mg of vitamin C or ascorbic acid daily. Note that vitamin C can also lower zinc levels, and zinc levels can be low in those who have CKD, particularly in the setting of a low-protein diet. If you are not eating a healthy diet, you may need to increase the levels of vitamin C in your diet, but do so only under a doctor's supervision.

Vitamin D

There are millions of people with low levels of vitamin D in this country—all ages, shapes, and sizes are affected. The combination of a lack of adequate sun exposure and a Western diet low in vitamin D is causing this nationwide deficiency. *Vitamin D deficiency is not found only in those with CKD, but also in those with normal kidney function.* And there are many whose vitamin D levels are dangerously low.

To clarify, there are two different types of vitamin D. The first type of vitamin D concerns vitamin D before it is further processed in the kidneys (the kidney-specific vitamin D we already spoke about in earlier chapters). Many people with CKD can be on *both* forms of vitamin D.

In addition to aiding bone health, vitamin D may have beneficial effects on the heart, as well as improve anemia and help the immune system. It may also help lower proteinuria. Vitamin D may potentially do a lot more and it is currently being researched.

Your doctor can order blood work to see what your vitamin D levels are. If they are low, two different types of replacement can be used. There is vitamin D2 and vitamin D3. Either form can be used, although the vitamin D3 is better absorbed. In general, your doctor may ask you to take one tablet, or 1000 IUs (International Units), of vitamin D3. Your doctor will then obtain follow-up blood work and depending on the test results, may change your dosage.

Vitamin E

Vitamin E is a very good antioxidant and some laboratory studies have demonstrated that it may help reduce oxidative stress and

inflammation in the kidneys. It may also reduce free radical formation and help reduce proteinuria in certain types of nephritis. Additionally, vitamin E may work well with alphalipoic acid for a more
significant anti-inflammatory effect.

The optimal dosage of vitamin E is not yet known. Given the
oxidative stress and inflammation present in CKD, a dose of 200 to
400 IUs may be beneficial. If you have nephritis, you may benefit
from a higher dose. Talk with your doctor before taking any vitamin
E, especially if you are on blood thinners. Further study is needed.

Vitamin K2

Vitamin K is often found in standard multivitamin and calcium supplements. If you have ever wondered what vitamin K is and why it
is important, you have come to the right place. There are a couple of
different forms of vitamin K. Most doctors and patients are familiar
with vitamin K1, which is a vitamin that is important in the body's
clotting system. When you are deficient in this vitamin, it can cause
a thinning of the blood. This is also how warfarin sodium (Coumadin),
an extremely popular blood thinner, acts. Often those on Coumadin
are advised to keep their intake of leafy green vegetables steady, as
any change in the amount you eat can affect vitamin K levels and
may require a change in Coumadin dosage.

Vitamin K2, on the other hand, is a vitamin that acts on bone;
specifically, it has been demonstrated to improve bone strength in
patients with osteoporosis. It also may have a protective effect on blood
vessels by inhibiting calcium build up on the walls of the vessels. If you
are taking Coumadin, it is not recommended that you take vitamin K2.

In many of the studies done with vitamin K2, high doses were
used. It needs more study in patients with advanced CKD, but a
dosage of 40 to 80 micrograms a day seems to be a reasonable starting amount.

OTHER NUTRITIONAL SUPPLEMENTS

In addition to vitamins, nutritional supplements are also beneficial.
Again, the optimal dosage of many of these supplements is not

known, although many are being studied. Talk with your physician regarding the dosages that are right for you.

Coenzyme Q$_{10}$

Coenzyme Q$_{10}$ is well known not only for its importance in different body systems, especially heart and cellular health, but also for its antioxidant role. One study suggested that it has significant antioxidant properties in kidney disease, but this needs to be further researched. Coenzyme Q$_{10}$ comes in various doses, but one should start at 50 to 100 mg and increase slowly.

Potassium and Magnesium

In the setting of kidney disease, your doctor will be checking your blood work to see if potassium or magnesium supplementation is needed. In advanced stages of kidney disease, however, supplementation is not recommended. The danger of high potassium and high magnesium levels to your body was discussed in previous chapters.

Calcium

Calcium supplementation in kidney disease is very complex and depends on several factors, including your medical situation and your phosphorus, vitamin D, PTH, and calcium levels as measured in the blood.

A normal calcium level in the blood is normally between 8.5 and 10. If your levels are lower than 8.5, your doctor may ask you to take additional calcium. Your doctor may also change the type of phosphorus binder that you are on depending on your calcium level.

There are many different types of calcium, with calcium carbonate and calcium citrate being the most common forms of replacement.

Alpha Lipoic Acid (ALA)

The ALA supplement is a potent antioxidant and is used not only for its ability to reduce oxidative stress, but also for its ability to replenish glutathione, which is another potent antioxidant in the body. Glu-

The Purity of Calcium Supplements

There was a major article published recently that looked at the lead content of many forms of calcium, both natural and synthetic. The study found that many types of calcium had measurable amounts of lead in them.

As consumers, you have many options when buying over-the-counter supplements. There are some types of calcium that have higher amounts of lead and traces of other metals in them. Certain natural forms, such as dolomite and bone meal, may have high levels of lead, whereas calcium carbonate, a popular type of calcium used by many healthcare professionals, was found to have minute, almost undetectable concentrations of lead. You need to be aware of what exactly you are purchasing, as it likely won't be on the label. The website www.consumerlab.com can help you navigate through different varieties.

tathione plays a major role in the elimination of certain toxins in the body and helps the immune system operate at an optimal level. Studies suggest that ALA may also have an antioxidant effect on the kidneys, especially in diabetic nephropathy. It has been especially studied in patients with diabetes-related nerve damage. Used with vitamin E, it may have an additional potent antioxidant effect.

There are different dosages for ALA. An optimal dose has not yet been established, but a minimal dose of 50 to 100 mg may be beneficial.

Omega-3 Supplements

Omega-3 fatty acids are not made by the body so therefore, they need to be obtained from dietary sources or supplements. A common form of supplementation is in fish oil. Omega-3 has been shown to have anti-inflammatory properties that can help many medical conditions, including heart disease and diabetes. There is also a role for omega-3 in the treatment of high cholesterol, particularly if high triglycerides are present.

With regards to kidney disease, the results have not been as encouraging. Studies looked at the role of omega-3 fatty acids in the treatment of IgA nephropathy, a type of nephritis. While high doses did not lower proteinuria, they did reduce oxidative stress. In other studies concerning other types of nephritis, it showed a possible effect on decreasing protein levels in the urine.

We are just beginning to learn about how inflammation affects the kidneys. There are likely several mechanisms that contribute to the level of inflammation in kidney disease, as spoken of in earlier chapters. With our Western diet, many of us do not consume enough omega-3. Supplementation of omega-3 and polyunsaturated fatty acids may not only reduce the inflammatory response in the kidneys and help prevent worsening of kidney function; it may also reduce the risk of coronary heart disease in those with CKD. The optimal dose of omega-3 supplementation is not known, but it may be higher doses than have been previously studied.

Omega-3 fatty acids are really the combination of two fatty acids called eicosapentaenoic acid (EPA) and docosahexaenoic acid (DPA). The ratio of EPA to DPA in a formulation may be important, as it is suggested that different ratios of these two in different formulations may give a different anti-inflammatory effect. There is an FDA-approved omega-3 medication called Lovaza for the treatment of high triglycerides. There are other forms that you can buy, as well, but no matter which you choose, it is important that it is mercury-free. Many will come in doses of either 1000 mg or 1200 mg. Normal dosage is two to three tablets a day, but can be higher depending on the inflammatory condition and triglyceride levels. Talk with your doctor before starting supplementation if you are taking any type of blood thinner.

Spirulina

Spirulina is an algae that likely has protective effects on the kidneys. It has a tremendous effect on lowering cholesterol and triglyceride levels, as it did in one study that looked at people with nephrotic syndrome. It may also help in lowering blood pressure.

There is no standard dosage for this supplement. Based on some studies, the usual dosage has been 500 to 1000 mg a day. It can interact with a number of blood pressure medications and diabetes medications, however, so consult with your doctor before taking it.

SUMMARY

Vitamins and natural supplements can play a significant role in kidney health. The full potential of many of these supplements still needs to be studied. Talk with your doctor before changing any aspect of your nutritional program.

12

Herbs & Complementary Therapies

Many herbal therapies have tremendous health and healing benefits. In fact, the National Institutes of Health (NIH) has a research section focused on herbal, alternative, and complementary medicine. If you are thinking about using herbs or herbal supplements and have chronic kidney disease, you need to be watchful concerning which supplements you decide to take. You should talk with your nephrologist before trying any new herbal supplement.

CONSIDERATIONS IN CHRONIC KIDNEY DISEASE

Having CKD means that you need to pay attention to the dosage of all medications. Whether it is a prescribed medication from your doctor or an herbal supplement, it can still enter the bloodstream and have toxic effects on the body. The worse the kidney function, the higher the risk.

All prescribed medications are regulated by the Food and Drug Administration (FDA), so you know you can always count on the ingredients being listed. There is, however, no current regulation of many herbal products, so many of their ingredients are unknown. Please understand I am not saying that more can't be done to improve the safety of prescribed medications. All I am saying is that we currently do not know the specific contents of several herbal preparations, and without any guidelines, the safety and efficacy of many these preparations is unknown.

If you are deciding on an herbal preparation, you need first educate yourself on potential interactions with your prescription medications. Most medications and other supplements are metabolized by the liver and filtered by the kidneys. Certain herbs and medications can affect the liver's processing of other medications, either slowing down their metabolism or speeding it up. Depending on the medication involved, this may be very harmful. Patients with kidney disease, especially at the advanced stages, are more susceptible to these changes as they have limited kidney reserve to begin with. Talk with your doctor and other health professionals before taking an herbal preparation, especially if you advanced kidney disease

COMMONLY USED HERBAL SUPPLEMENTS

In this section, you will read about common herbal supplements that are being used for kidney disease. Keep in mind that the following list contains only a summary of commonly prescribed herbs; it is only intended to be used as a guide. Do not begin any of these supplements without first talking with your nephrologist and other health care providers.

Alfalfa

A great source of vitamins and some minerals, alfalfa has been used in the treatment of diabetes and fluid retention. However, this supplement may actually increase the level of inflammation in the body. In one study, primates given alfalfa developed a condition that mimicked lupus. In another, it caused a syndrome in monkeys that again resembled lupus. CKD is an inflammatory condition itself, and the fact that alfalfa can have that kind of effect on the immune system warrants further study in those with CKD, especially if any type of nephritis is involved.

There is no standard alfalfa dosage, but some experts use it at doses of greater than 300 mg three times a day. Alfalfa can also be given in a tea form. Be careful if you are on a blood thinner like Coumadin, as alfalfa contains vitamin K. And in general, be careful if you insist on using this particular supplement.

Aloe

Aloe is used to treat many conditions, including stomach ulcers and colitis. That being said, it can sometimes cause diarrhea and affect kidney function, as well as affect electrolyte levels, including potassium. There have been some reported cases of kidney failure that were felt to be caused by aloe. Avoid using it if you have kidney disease.

Astragalus

Astragalus has been studied in treating different forms of the nephrotic syndrome and has shown promising results. In two different studies, it was effective at significantly lowering the protein levels in the urine. In may be even be effective for the many different causes of proteinuria. In a laboratory-based study, it showed benefit in reducing the levels of protein in early diabetes nephropathy. For people who are on potent medications that lower the immune system, it may help reduce the risk of infection, as well. Further study is needed, but this herb has great potential in the treatment of nephritis and in lowering proteinuria.

The optimal dosage of astragalus is not yet known. In the one report, the dosage was started at 15 g per day. The dosage is important because different amounts may have different effects on the immune system. It also depends if you are using the root or the extract. Further study is needed, but astragalus seems to have many healing benefits.

N-Acetylcysteine (NAC)

NAC has traditionally been used for the treatment of acetaminophen drug overdose. It is also given to most people with CKD before going for any type of imaging study or procedure involving the use of contrast dye. A potent antioxidant and anti-inflammatory drug, NAC has been studied for the treatment of other forms of nephritis, as well. There is actually a clinical research trial to be done that is examining NAC and another herbal supplement, milk thistle, for the treatment of diabetic nephropathy. Go to www.clinicaltrials.gov for more information.

The optimal dose for NAC is not known at this point. However, in studies looking at the kidneys' protective effects before having any contrast dye-related study, the minimum dose was 600 mg twice daily. Doses of 600 to 1200 mg twice daily are generally safe with only mild nausea and stomach upset as common side effects. It also has a rather unpleasant smell that can make it intolerable to some people. An interesting question regarding NAC is whether long-term use can protect the kidneys over months or even years. It has excellent potential, but more studies are needed.

Buchu

Buchu is used to help treat water retention and urinary tract infections, but it may irritate and be toxic to the kidneys. Buchu is not to be used at all if you have kidney disease.

Corn Silk

Corn silk is used to treat kidney and bladder infections. It is also used for water retention and it may lower potassium levels. However, be careful of using it in CKD, because both kidney function and electrolyte levels can be affected.

The optimal dosage for corn silk is not known, but it is suggested that as little as 4 g can be made into a tea. Whether this dose has to be reduced for kidney disease is not known.

Cranberry

Cranberry has been shown to be of benefit in the prevention of urinary tract infections, and it may also decrease the risks of kidney stones that are associated with urinary tract infections. It has minimal side effects and people generally tolerate it very well.

Cranberry can be taken in several forms, including capsules or juice. To prevent urinary tract infections, a common recommendation is 10 to 15 ounces of pure cranberry juice daily. Another option is two take two, 300 or 400 mg capsules daily.

Dandelion Root

Dandelion root is used for the treatment of infections of the urinary tract. It works like a diuretic and has some anti-inflammation and anti-oxidant activity. It can also have an effect on lowering blood pressure. As it contains potassium, I would hesitate to use dandelion root in advanced CKD given the risk of high potassium and dehydration.

There are various dosage regimens and ways to administer dandelion root, including capsule form. It is unknown if the dose needs to be adjusted for kidney disease, but I would use the lowest dose possible. Avoid using this if you have stage three CKD or greater, given the possible effects just listed.

Garlic

Garlic is use to treat a wide variety of conditions, from hypertension to diabetes. Because it has strong antioxidant properties, it is has been utilized in the treatment of cancer and other inflammatory diseases. It is not surprising that there are laboratory-based studies showing that garlic may also help protect the kidneys. It seems to be able to reduce the levels of lead and other heavy metals in the body, as well.

Garlic comes in many forms, including tablets, a powdered form and the bulb itself. In kidney disease, the optimal dose of garlic is not yet known. Some studies suggest that high doses can worsen the function of the kidneys and other organs. It is the lower doses that seem to have the antioxidant effect. I would suggest starting with the garlic extract tablets at a low dose of 100 to 200 mg daily. Given the overabundance of toxins and heavy metals in the water, garlic may offer an additional protective effect on the kidneys by reducing the concentration of lead and other heavy metals in them. This needs to be studied more, but I would support a low daily dose of garlic.

Ginseng

There are two types of ginseng: American and Asian. The Asian form is more processed and is preferred by consumers. Ginseng is used to treat a number of conditions, including diabetes and fluid retention. There are several laboratory-based studies showing that ginseng may also have a protective effect on the kidneys. Additionally, heat-processed ginseng seems to have a protective effect in diabetic nephropathy. It may have antioxidant properties as well, but more study is needed.

Ginseng can be given in several forms, including capsules and tea bags. The optimal dose in kidney disease is not yet known. Some herbalists recommend 0.4 to 0.5 g once or twice daily. However, because large doses can be toxic to the body and interact with many medications used for diabetes and certain antidepressants, I would suggest starting with the lowest possible dose of 100 mg daily, and slowly increasing from there. Given the potential for many significant drug interactions, I would talk with your doctor before starting this herbal supplement.

Goldenrod

Goldenrod has many uses, including treatment of certain types of kidney stones, fluid retention, and inflammatory processes in the kidneys. The optimal dosage is not known in kidney disease, and I would not recommend using this supplement in kidney disease until further studies are done.

Green Tea

Green tea is a potent antioxidant and has been to treat many health problems from arthritis to cancer. A laboratory-based study suggests that it may also decrease the level of inflammation in people who have hypertension and diabetes, although further testing is needed.

Green tea is relatively safe and comes as either a tea bag or in capsule form. If you have high blood pressure, be aware that there is caffeine in green tea. Because caffeine has diuretic properties, be careful if you are on a prescribed diuretic.

Hawthorn

Hawthorn is very effective at treating both high blood pressure and congestive heart failure. It comes in many forms, but the easiest way to dose is to take capsules, usually 250 to 500 mg, twice daily to start. There is not any dosage changes required in kidney disease, but monitor your blood pressure closely if you are on this medication.

Juniper Oil

Juniper has been used to treat various ailments, including high blood pressure and arthritis. However, if you have kidney disease, do not take this herb. It can worsen kidney function.

Licorice

Licorice is used to treat stomach problems, ulcers, and many other ailments. Side effects can include raised blood pressure, edema, and a lowering of potassium. An optimal dose in kidney disease has not yet been established. If you have CKD, I would definitely avoid taking this supplement.

Milk Thistle

Much research has been done on the beneficial effects of milk thistle on liver disease, and new studies are looking at its possible beneficial effects in kidney disease. There is currently a National Institute of Health (NIH)-sponsored study that will examine the role of milk thistle and NAC in diabetic nephropathy.

The optimal dose of milk thistle has not yet been established. If you use capsules, some herbalists recommend starting at doses of around 400 mg taken twice daily. Again, I would recommend starting low, at 50 to 100 mg once or twice daily, and gradually increasing the dose.

Noni Juice

Noni juice contains a lot of potassium. In someone with CKD, this supplement should be avoided.

Parsley

Parsley is used to treat many conditions, including edema and high blood pressure. It has also been used to treat kidney stones, urinary tract infections, and GI tract symptoms. However, high doses of this supplement may worsen kidney function, as well as increase swelling and raise blood pressure.

The parsley leaf is commonly used as a garnish and is relatively safe. But if you have kidney disease, be careful when using the parsley oil or parsley seeds. I would recommend not using this medication if you have advanced kidney disease.

Pomegranate

Pomegranate juice has many properties and uses. It has beneficial effects concerning cholesterol and also lowers blood pressure, both of which are risk factors for worsening kidney disease. Pomegranate juice does contain potassium, however, and it can affect the liver, although further study is needed.

The optimal dose of pomegranate is not yet known. It is also not known if pomegranate can affect the kidneys in the same way as ACE inhibitors, especially in advanced stages where high potassium can be a significant problem. I would not suggest taking it if you have advanced kidney disease or problems with high potassium. If you are on ACE inhibitors/ARBS, or other medications that can raise potassium, I would avoid using this herb.

Turmeric

Turmeric is a very potent antioxidant that has been used to treat many conditions, including cancer. The active ingredient, curcumin, has been used for centuries. In some laboratory-based studies, it has been shown to have a strong anti-inflammatory effect on the kidneys. It may block the effects of TGF-beta on the kidneys, as well.

The optimal dose of turmeric is still not known. If you are taking curcumin, herbalists recommend taking 400 mg two to three times a day. With CKD, I recommend starting with a very low dose and watching the interaction with other prescription medications. Further study is needed.

TOXINS AND THE KIDNEYS

All of us live in a very toxic environment. You have most likely already read about the toxins—including heavy metals—in our water supply and their effects on kidney function. Additionally, think about the damaging effects of many of the processed foods, chemicals, and pesticides that we put into our bodies. Also consider the consequence of increased oxidative stress and the inflammatory response of high blood pressure, diabetes, and obesity on the kidneys.

Our kidneys are bombarded by the effects of this toxic buildup every day. Therefore, there should be a role for toxin removal to improve our kidney health. With the kidneys, however, you need to be careful.

The Process of Detoxification

If your body cannot get rid of the toxins it encounters, it makes sense that you will feel ill, exhausted, irritable, and lethargic. No one wants that, so detoxification becomes beneficial. Detoxification is the process of removing harmful toxins from the body.

Many excellent detoxification formulas are mixtures of several different herbal supplements. In addition to herbs, many cleanses can also contain vitamins and minerals, and many are diuretics that stimulate urination. There are detoxification formulas just for the kidneys and combination formulas for more than one body system. Examples of this are the combination liver and kidney detoxification formulas.

The Effect of Detoxification on Kidney Function

Under supervision by a qualified practitioner, detoxification is an excellent way to bring your body into balance *if you have normal kidney function*. There are several reasons I emphasize this. With CKD, especially in the advanced stages, the excessive urination and risk of dehydration associated with detoxification can affect kidney function. Such forced urination may increase the workload of the kidney. Additionally, your kidneys are receiving the combined effects of all the herbs in the cleansing formula at one time, many of which contain potassium, like juniper and dandelion root. With diabetes and advanced CKD, the kidneys can have difficulty getting rid of this often harmful extra potassium load.

Another concern about detoxification and kidney function is the required time. The time commitment to various detoxification programs is different. Some are short, lasting only one to three days; others can be as long as thirty days. In CKD, doing a rapid detoxification may actually worsen kidney function. The kidneys are very sensitive to rapid fluid changes in the body. With the "kidney flushing" properties of many of these rapid formulas, the risks of dehydration, electrolyte imbalances, and worsening kidney function are significant. I would avoid doing any type of rapid detoxification if CKD is present. If you have stage 1 or stage 2 kidney disease and you choose to do a rapid detoxification, I would do so under the close supervision of your nephrologist or complementary health care provider.

A slower detoxification process—one that is more kidney-friendly—may be an acceptable alternative. If your doctor does not have you on any type of fluid restriction, I would recommend drinking a lot of purified, alkalinized water. In addition, the use of certain teas, such as green tea, can be helpful because it is a natural diuretic.

By doing a more gradual detox, you have a much lower risk of developing dehydration and worsening kidney function. This approach is less traumatic to the kidneys and it will improve how you feel over time. In addition, add a glass of freshly juiced vegetables daily. Equally as important is eating fruits and vegetables that are abundant in antioxidants. It doesn't make any sense to detoxify if you are not going to change your eating habits.

Consider Liver Cleanses

Many of the available liver cleanses contain ingredients that are either kidney protective or kidney beneficial, including the vitamins

B_1, B_6, B_{12}, E, folic acid, N-acetylcysteine, and milk thistle—the last two of which are currently being studied for their kidney protective benefits. I would look for a cleanse that contained all or most of these, although a better option would be to take the ingredients separately. Before attempting any type of cleansing program, however, *first consult with your doctor.*

PROBIOTICS AND KIDNEY DISEASE

Your intestines are filled with "good bacteria" whose job is to help in the digestion of food and maintain balance by preventing the growth of "bad bacteria." When we take antibiotics, we disrupt the normal balance in the intestines, because the medicine can wipe out both good and bad bacteria. Probiotics are good bacteria that we put back into our bodies to restore and maintain balance in the intestines. A common way to take this is via a dietary supplement, and there are many of them out there.

In addition to maintaining balance, probiotics may have a role in kidney disease. The intestines and the kidneys both have a role in processing the toxins that can build up in kidney disease. In advanced CKD, the use of probiotics may improve the processing and removal of toxins. One example is a probiotic supplement from Kibow Biotech. For more information about this, you can refer to their website at www.kibowbiotech.com. More research is needed in this area, but it represents a new area of treatment for CKD. Again, talk with your doctor and other health providers before trying any new medication or dietary supplement.

COMPLEMENTARY AND ALTERNATIVE THERAPIES

Complementary therapies are being researched and used in combination with Western Medicine more and more each day. I don't like the term complementary because it implies that this treatment is separate and should be treated as such. Many physicians are using the term "integrated" instead, which I think is much better word. An integrated approach that uses all forms of available and relevant therapies is the best approach. If you decide to utilize any of the therapies described below, it should be done under the close supervision of both your kidney doctor and qualified health practitioner.

Osteopathy and Osteopathic Manipulative Medicine (OMM)

There is no better example of an integrated approach to medicine than osteopathy. It is a practice of medicine that focuses on treating the whole person, not just a particular illness. I am one of many osteopathic physicians. We are trained not only in "Western" medicine, but also in using the healing power of touch to treat illness— osteopathic manipulative medicine (OMM). The founder of osteopathy, Andrew Taylor Still, recognized the important role of a "hands-on" approach in treating people. Therefore, all osteopathic physicians are trained in the basics of OMM in medical school; some even undergo further specialized training to become practitioners solely in OMM.

Through the use of different types of manipulative techniques, including *myofascial (my-o-fash-el)* techniques—a type of muscle massage—OMM is used in the treatment of many illnesses, including hypertension. There are other techniques that are utilized specifically for the treatments of edema as well. I believe that touch is an essential component of the healing process and OMM is a great example of this. Please see the Resources section for more information (page 161).

Chiropractic Medicine

This is a great form of hands-on medicine that focuses on the spine and spinal mechanics as a cause and contribution to health and disease. There is an overlap with chiropractic care and OMM, as many people benefit from their expertise with an improvement in overall health and well-being. With regards to high blood pressure and kidney disease, if the spine is not in line, it can alter the character of the nerves that affect blood pressure and the kidneys. This increased "sympathetic tone" of the nerves can increase the blood pressure and affect kidney blood flow. Both chiropractic medicine and OMM can restore the body to its natural balance through different, but complementary forms of therapy.

Acupuncture

Acupuncture is an ancient practice that, like OMM, has a beneficial effect on the whole body. More specifically, it may have an anti-inflammatory effect on the body and may be beneficial in kidney disease. More studies are certainly needed, but I think some preliminary evidence suggests acupuncture may have an effect on lowering blood pressure as well.

Homeopathy

In contrast to Western medicine, the approach of homeopathy is that less is more. In other words, very small quantities of medicine can have significant effects on healing. The risk of experiencing toxic effects to any medication in homeopathy is slim to none. More study is needed in the use of homeopathy for the treatment of kidney disease. See the Resources section for more information (page 161).

Chelation

Chelation (kee-lay-shun) is a treatment for purifying the blood that effectively removes toxins and other pollutants, including heavy metals, from the body. It has also been used in treating clogged blood vessels, diabetes, and heart disease—research is ongoing regarding chelation and heart disease.

As discussed in prior chapters, lead and other heavy metals that we are exposed to can worsen kidney disease. The effect of heavy metals on kidney disease is a lot more common than we think. In an important study, chelation improved kidney function in people with a long-term, low-level exposure to lead.

Chelation treatment involves administering a "chelating agent" called EDTA (chemical name: ethylenedinitrilo-tetraacetic acid) through a vein (intravenously). This agent can also be given in a pill form. There are natural forms of chelation, as well. Medications in pill form used for chelation can include EDTA, vitamin C, garlic, and other natural agents. Watch the dose and type of agent you decide to use. Some of the oral forms may have high potassium and magnesium levels. Talk with your doctor if you are deciding on this form of therapy, as blood work needs to be monitored closely. There are many potential benefits of chelation therapy that need to be further studied.

Meditative Therapies

In Chapter 9, we talked at length about the importance of meditation and stress reduction. I cannot emphasize enough how important this is, not only to reduce anxiety, but also to lower stress, improve blood pressure, and improve one's well-being.

SUMMARY

For many of the conditions we discussed in the preceding chapters, a combination approach to treatment is the best approach. In diabetic nephropathy, for example, in addition to using ACE inhibitors/ARBS, the use of vitamins, antioxidants, and certain herbal supplements can be beneficial. More research is needed, however, to establish what the optimal dosage is.

13

$\int$piritual and Emotional Components of Healing

W hat is the essence of a human being? This question has been asked by many throughout history, including philosophers and theologians. As human beings, we are more than the sum of our parts—we are spiritual. We have feelings, fears, beliefs, and needs, and our spiritual and emotional aspects are integral to the healing process.

This book has been a journey—each chapter a stepping-stone to broaden your knowledge of kidney disease and provide you with the tools you need to improve your physical well-being. This last chapter, however, focuses on intangible qualities that are equally as important to the healing process as the physical component. In order to improve your health, you have to want to do it and have the belief that you *can* do it. It is that belief, that faith, that enables you to take that very important first step to getting better.

THE POWER OF CONNECTION

None of us are islands unto ourselves. We are connected with everything and everyone around us. Our bodies remain in balance because of the constant communication between all of our body systems and cells. Having an illness, especially one that requires hospitalization, is a time of extreme disconnection physically, emotionally, and spiritually. The illness not only causes imbalance and disharmony in the body, but the isolation from family and loved ones can also invoke feelings of despair. These negative feelings can hurt the healing process.

Norman Cousins, in his book *Anatomy of an Illness as Perceived by the Patient,* said "The inevitable question arose in my mind: what about the positive emotions? If negative emotions produce negative chemical changes in the body, wouldn't the positive emotions produce positive chemical changes? Is it possible that love, hope, faith, laughter, confidence, and the will to live have therapeutic value? Do chemical changes occur only on the downside?"

When we feel connected, we change. We become more positive, more invigorated. People do better when family members and friends are present. I always request, if possible, that a family member be present when talking with a patient. Not only do they function as an extra set of eyes and ears concerning the medical aspects of care, but more importantly, they serve as a support system, a rock. People with CKD, especially in the advanced stages, are on an emotional and physical roller coaster due to the nature of the disease. Illness is a humbling experience for anybody, and no one should have to go through it alone.

THE POWER OF PRAYER

Many of us experience a need to feel connected with something higher than ourselves. While the connection with family and friends is important, this higher, spiritual connection is also vital in the healing process.

One night while on call, I was asked to urgently see a man who was very ill in the emergency room. He had a debilitating pneumonia, his blood pressure was low, he was in a state of shock, and his kidney function was worsening. He was so critically ill that he was soon transferred to the intensive care unit.

I went out to the waiting area to meet with his family and it was a positive but overwhelming experience. They were holding hands and were engaged in a communal prayer. When they finished, I introduced myself and explained to them the nature of their family member's illness. I was flabbergasted when they asked me to join them in prayer. I held hands with the family as each murmured a small prayer of healing. When it was finished, I was hugged by several members of the family, and they asked me to pray each day for their loved one.

In those tense early days in the ICU when the patient's condition was grave—when the pneumonia that ravaged his body was so bad it was unclear if he would pull through—he was never left alone. There was always a family member present, praying with and for him. They all held his hand and whispered words of encouragement. When he was able to eat, they helped feed him. They were a constant source of encouragement, and each day when I visited they invited me to join them in prayer.

For a short time, the patient did need to be on dialysis. After several weeks, though, he recovered from the debilitating pneumonia and his kidney function slowly recovered. I am wholeheartedly convinced that without the support, encouragement, and prayer from his family, he would not have done as well.

Through that experience, I gained a new insight into the role of prayer. The role of this book is not to advocate for any specific religious practice or creed; rather, I am simply saying that I believe prayer is a way to connect with the spiritual side of human beings and aid in the healing process. Prayer gives the person and her family a significant motivation to get better and even further, addresses those intangibles I talked about that make us whole.

Studies examining the role that prayer has in affecting the healing process have been mixed, and it is a very difficult topic to research. In one study, prayer had an effect on the healing of wounds in primates. The group that was prayed for had better results in healing its wounds than did the other group. Additionally, the work of physicians like Dr. Larry Dossey and Dr. Mitchell Krucoff suggest that prayer can be effective. Other studies, however, have had conflicting results.

Studying the effect of prayer is very difficult; there is so much about prayer that we don't understand and more study needs to be done. That being said, I sincerely believe that it is an integral aspect of total care. When patients or their families ask, I pray with them. And if I visit someone in the hospital who is in the process praying or meeting with their pastor or spiritual adviser, I will wait until they are finished. Prayer should not be interrupted.

THE POWER OF LAUGHTER

In Norman Cousins' medical memoir, he wrote of how he used laughter as part of the healing process. Laughter is a great way to cope with anxiety and tension, and it can help maintain a positive attitude by relieving stress and improving mood. Additionally, it can help the physical healing process by lowering blood pressure and lowering blood sugars in those with diabetes. Given that these two conditions are responsible for the majority of kidney disease in this country, laughter and humor should be part of the healing process.

MUSIC AS A HEALING THERAPY

What is life without music? I know I could not imagine a life without it. Music has many healing qualities. It relaxes us, it can calm our fears, and it may help lower our blood pressure and improve our overall health, which makes complete sense given that all of us are musical. What do I mean by this? There is a musical rhythm to everything in our bodies. Our hearts quite literally, have their own musical rhythm.

While much has been described on the psychological effects of musical healing, it is also important to note that it has physical effects as well. A study was done in Canada concerning music therapy and those on dialysis. Music helped with relieving depression, relieving anxiety, and lowering stress levels. So go ahead. Turn up the radio!

THE SIX-DAY, FIVE-MINUTE START-UP PLAN

In the beginning of this chapter, the goal was to get you thinking about the way to better kidney and overall health. The journey of a thousand miles begins with a single step. Take that first step on the pathway to your health journey today. Gradually, you will acquire a new insight and be an ambassador for a healthy lifestyle; but for now, just try using this simple start-up plan.

The plan is like going up a set of stairs; each day you take another step up towards your goal. It may be a small step, but the important thing is to not go backwards. We never go down, we only go up. *Always up!*

Day One: Take a Five Minute Walk

All you need for this first step is a good pair of walking shoes and a commitment. The beauty of walking for exercise is that you can adapt the time and pace to fit your age and condition—all I am asking for is five minutes the first time out.

Keep a walking diary so that you can concretely see your progress. Try to increase your walks by a minute each time so that you are eventually walking for thirty minutes three to four times a week. In the event of cold or inclement weather, check out your neighborhood mall; most have an indoor walking program.

Day Two: Eat a Healthy Breakfast

It can be difficult to change your eating habits all at once. So, in this second step, I'm just asking you to change one meal at a time. Start with breakfast. Make it a priority each morning to put something healthy into your body. Whether it is a sprouted grain cereal, vegetable omelet, or something as simple as a glass of vegetable juice, make the commitment to that first meal of the day. A simple breakfast meal can take as little as five minutes. You will eventually find that a healthy lunch and dinner will fall into place, too.

Day Three: Take a Time Out

In our hectic worlds, we often make time for our spouses, children, parents, and friends, but none for ourselves. To complete step three, make daily relaxation for at least five minutes a priority. Learn relaxation techniques, such as deep breathing with your diaphragm, that you can do in five to ten minutes. These short intervals of meditative therapy can do a lot in keeping you centered and reducing the effects of every day stress. Make the commitment and take five minutes!

Day Four: Decrease Your Coffee or Soft Drink Intake By One

Think about a typical workday. There's probably coffee in the morning, a mid-morning coffee break, a soft drink for lunch, coffee in the mid-afternoon to help keep you awake after that heavy lunch, and coffee or a soft drink with dinner. Starting today, decrease the amount of coffee or soda you drink by one cup. The time it takes to buy it from the vendor and subsequently drink it is about five minutes. Use that five minutes for something else instead, like time for meditation. Continue reducing by one cup each week. Rome wasn't built in a day, and caffeine is something from which you will have to gradually wean yourself.

Day Five: Decrease The Amount You Smoke

Why do we smoke? For many of us, it is a great stress reliever. There is nothing like going out for that five minute smoke break. Think about how many smoke breaks you take daily. Maybe it is one when you wake up, one at work in the middle of the day, one late in the afternoon, and one at night before bed. That's a lot of five minutes. Take one less smoke break a week. Give yourself those five minutes back. If you are continuous chain smoker, reduce the amount you smoke by 5 percent each week. After several weeks, you may have an additional half-hour or whole hour back you didn't know you'd been missing.

Day Six: Get to Sleep Five Minutes Earlier

Now that you have been exercising more, you are likely more tired each night. For many of us, sleep is a priority we forget about. The solution is simple. Each week, go to sleep five minutes earlier. After six weeks of this, you will have gained a half-hour of sleep. If you can give yourself an additional half-hour to hour of sleep each night, you will be all the better for it. And all it takes is five minutes.

As you can see, this is a rather simple, yet ambitious plan. I assure you, though, it is very doable. It may be difficult at first, but that is why we are starting with small changes. Over time, the small steps will become a full flight of stairs. You will have walked to the top without even realizing it, and your kidneys will thank you.

SUMMARY

The healing process is not just a physical one. Beyond healing your body, you also need to heal your spirit. It is important to utilize all potential modes of healing that are available. Mind, body, and spirit are all connected.

Conclusion

This book has told you what you need to know about both kidney health and kidney disease. But knowing is just the first step; now you must *do*. While the diagnosis of kidney disease may have first made you feel helpless, you are now aware of all the steps you can take to greatly improve not only kidney function, but also overall well-being. You are far from helpless. In fact, an arsenal of health-promoting weapons is at your disposal.

Start by talking to your doctor so that you can ask relevant questions about your treatment plan—questions that will yield the information you need to make smart decisions. Make the all-important dietary modifications that can slow or even halt the progression of your disorder. Consider complementary therapies, from acupuncture to herbal supplementation, that can improve the function of your whole body. Spend time forging stronger family ties and spiritual bonds. Every positive step you take will not only make your body stronger, but also make each individual day more enjoyable and rewarding.

And at the risk of sounding cliché, I want to remind you that just because you have kidney disease doesn't mean it has to have you. This book has put the power of change in your hands, and I urge you to be proactive in your search for greater health. If you have further questions or you just want to fill me in on your progress, please look for my website, www.kidneyrescuemission.com. I look forward to hearing from you.

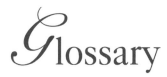

Glossary

The following terms are often used in discussions of kidney function and disease. By becoming familiar with them, you will be able to have more productive discussions with your healthcare provider and also be better able to understand printed information on this subject.

acidosis. An imbalance in the body caused by either a buildup of acid or loss of bicarbonate. Kidney disease can increase the acid levels in the body.

acute kidney failure (AKF). A worsening of kidney function occurring over a few days to a few weeks. Blood work showing a rise in the serum creatinine or a reduction in the GFR (glomerular filtration rate) is used to confirm AKF.

anemia. A deficiency of red blood cells or hemoglobin, the oxygen-carrying pigment in the blood. This condition can be determined through blood work.

chronic kidney disease (CKD). A worsening of kidney function over a period of a few weeks to a few months. The severity of chronic kidney disease is expressed in terms of five stages, with stage five being the most serious.

contrast-induced kidney failure. The worsening of kidney function one to two days after an imaging study—like a CAT scan—or an interventional procedure in which dye is used. If such a study is needed, there are measures that can be taken prior to the procedure to help the kidneys.

creatinine. A waste product of muscle metabolism that is measured to determine kidney function and to calculate glomerular filtration rate (GFR).

cytokine. A type of protein that, as part of the immune system, can stimulate and perpetuate inflammation.

diabetic nephropathy. A condition, caused by long-standing diabetes mellitus, that is the most common cause of kidney disease in the United States. Diabetic nephropathy can be detected through a special type of urine protein test.

dialysis. An artificial filtering process that cleans and purifies the blood when the kidneys are no longer able to do so.

edema. Swelling in the feet, ankles, legs, or eyes due to an accumulation of fluids. Edema can be sign of kidney disease or of problems with heart and liver function.

glomerular filtration rate (GFR). A measure of kidney function and stage of kidney disease based on the level of creatinine, a waste product of muscle metabolism.

glomerulonephritis (GN). A type of kidney disease characterized by inflammation of the glomeruli, which are small blood vessels found in the kidneys.

hematuria. The presence of blood in the urine. Many conditions, including kidney stones, nephritis, and cancer, can cause this disorder.

inflammation. An immune system response to trauma, disease, or illness, that is characterized by pain and swelling. In certain circumstances, the inflammatory process is never turned off, which, over time, can have damaging effects on the kidneys and other body organs.

interstitial nephritis. A kidney disorder in which the spaces between the kidney tubules become inflamed. This disorder can have many causes, including certain medications.

macroscopic hematuria. Blood in the urine that can be seen with the naked eye.

microscopic hematuria. Blood in the urine that can be seen only through use of a microscope.

nephritis. Inflammation of the kidneys.

nephrotic syndrome (NS). A syndrome characterized by severe edema (accumulation of fluids in the tissue) and large amounts of protein in the urine.

parathyroid hormone. A hormone that regulates calcium and phosphorus concentrations in the body, thereby having an effect on both bone and kidney health.

polycystic kidney disease (PKD). A common inherited condition that causes cysts to form in the kidneys and sometimes the liver.

proteinuria. The presence of protein in the urine. This condition, a sign of kidney disease, can be determined through a simple urine test.

renin-angiotensin-aldosterone (RAA) system. A hormone system that regulates blood pressure and fluid balance. Problems with this system can worsen inflammation and adversely affect kidney function.

sleep apnea. An abnormal sleep pattern characterized by pauses in breathing that can last several seconds or longer. Sleep apnea is a common cause of resistant hypertension, a specific type of high blood pressure.

transforming growth factor (TGF) beta. A type of toxic protein believed to be responsible for the continued inflammatory response associated with many chronic diseases, including chronic kidney disease.

uremia. An accumulation of nitrogenous wastes (urea) in the blood that occurs during end-stage kidney disease (kidney function of less than 10 percent). Symptoms can include, but are not limited to, nausea, dry heaves, vomiting, and extreme fatigue.

Resources

The Internet provides easy access to further information on kidney disease, qualified healthcare providers, complementary therapies, nutrition, and more. The websites listed below are a great place to start, but be aware that new and helpful sites are being created all the time to serve people with kidney disease and their families.

INFORMATIVE WEBSITES ON KIDNEY DISEASE

American Association of Kidney Patients

The American Association of Kidney Patients (AAKP) is a national non-profit organization—founded by kidney patients for kidney patients—that is dedicated to helping those on hemodialysis and peritoneal dialysis, as well as those who have received transplants. Its website provides extensive information on kidney disease and related subjects, offers helpful magazines and newsletters, and lists links to other valuable sites.
Website: www.aakp.org

American Kidney Fund

This is a national organization that not only helps fight kidney disease through education, but also provides monetary aid to those victims of kidney disease who require it. Last year they were able to provide financial support to one out of every five patients on dialysis. Donations can be made online by clicking the "Give Now" tab on the opening page of their website.
Website: www.kidneyfund.org

National Kidney Foundation

The National Kidney Foundation is dedicated to preventing kidney and urinary tract disorders, improving the health and well-being of individuals and families affected by kidney disease, and increasing the availability of organs for transplantation. Visit the foundation's website for information on diet, dialysis, medication, transplantation, and more. If you are interested in free kidney evaluation screenings, click on "Kidney Disease," then "KEEP Early Detection Screenings," then "Find a KEEP Screening Near You."
Website: www.kidney.org

Nephrology Channel

Set up in a style similar to that of traditional news websites, the Nephrology Channel provides related breaking news headlines, health reports, newsletters, and more. This is a great place to remain in-the-know about current nephrology news, discoveries, and trends.
Website: www.nephrologychannel.com

Polycystic Kidney Disease Foundation

The Polycystic Kidney Disease (PKD) Foundation was formed in 1982 for the purpose of fighting PKD through research, education, advocacy, support, and awareness. Visit this website to stay current on related news, connect with your local chapter, advocate to your local officials, and more. Click on "Learn" for information on kidney disease, or on "Research" to read about clinical trials and studies.
Website: www.pkdcure.org

FINDING COMPLEMENTARY HEALTH PROVIDERS AND THERAPIES

American Board of Integrative Holistic Medicine

The goal of the American Board of Integrative Holistic Medicine is to train doctors to work with patients towards wellness. Click on the "Patients" tab and then on "Locate Certified Physicians" to find a board-certified holistic physician in your area.
Website: www.holisticboard.org

American Massage Therapy Association

The mission of the American Massage Therapy Association is to serve its members while advancing the art, science, and practice of massage therapy. To find a therapist near you, click on the "Find a Massage Therapist" tab, fill in your name and location, and check the boxes of the services in which you are interested.
Website: www.amtamassage.org

ChiroWeb

ChiroWeb offers alternative medical news, information, and research breakthroughs. Visit its discussion forum, watch one of its many webcasts, or simply use it as a way to locate a local chiropractor who has the specific training and expertise for which you are looking
Website: www.chiroweb.com

National Center for Homeopathy

The National Center for Homeopathy provides education for both the general public and homeopaths. In addition to its "Find a Homeopath" service, the website presents information on homeopathy and a range of health topics.
Website: www.homeopathic.org

The National Center on Physical Activity and Disability

Purposeful movement is an important part of kidney disease treatment, and water exercises provide a great alternative for those who have a hard time moving on land. To find an aquatic therapy service near you, visit this website, click on the link titled "Aquatic Therapy," and then click on "Organizations."
Website: www.ncpad.org/exercise/

National Certification Commission for Acupuncture and Oriental Medicine

The mission of the NCCAOM is to establish, assess, and promote recognized standards of competence and safety in acupuncture and oriental medicine. Click on the "Find a Practitioner" tab to locate practitioners who are nationally certified in oriental medicine, acupuncture, Chinese herbology, or Asian bodywork therapy.
Website: www.nccaom.org

FINDING TRADITIONAL MEDICAL DOCTORS

Doctors.At

Doctors.At allows you to browse for physicians by state and specialty. Complementary healthcare providers can also be located through this website.
Website: www.doctors.at

Health Grades

Health Grades guides you to physicians (including specialists), hospitals, nursing homes, and other healthcare resources in your area. It also provides ratings on prescription drugs.
Website: www.healthgrades.com

DRINKING WATER SAFETY INFORMATION

Local Drinking Water Information

This website of the Environmental Protection Agency (EPA) collects reports from public water systems across the country. Click on the appropriate area of the US map to see if your local water system has submitted a water quality report.
Website: www.epa.gov/safewater/dwinfo.htm

Water Filter Ratings

This page of the Consumer Search website provides information on water filters and offers links to reputable sources that have ranked various filters.
Website: www.consumersearch.com/water-filters/reviews

NUTRITIONAL INFORMATION AND DIET PLANS

Calorie Count

This website enables you to create a free account that offers personalized dietary tools, advice, and support. Also included is a nutrition blog, a question-and-answer forum, and nutritional information—including calorie counts—for a wide range of foods.
Website: www.caloriecount.com

The Daily Plate

The Daily Plate offers an easy, cost-free way to track what you eat each day. You begin by calculating your calorie goals. The website then guides you in achieving your ideal weight through healthy dietary habits.
Website: www.thedailyplate.com

DASH Diet

This page of the National Heart, Lung, and Blood Institute website presents the full DASH eating plan—a plan designed to prevent or reduce hypertension. Included are helpful dietary guidelines and full menus for breakfast, lunch, dinner, and snacks.
Website: www.nhlbi.nih.gov/health/public/heart/hbp/dash/new_dash.pdf

Glycemic Index

This website provides basic information on the glycemic index, answers common questions, and offers tips for switching to a low-glycemic index diet.
Website: www.glycemicindex.com

The Nephron Information Center Food Values

This site offers nutritional information sourced from the USDA. Simply type in the name of the food or a select a category, and get results. Do not

overlook the links to kidney-specific nutrition information, which are almost hidden at the top of the website.
Website: www.foodvalues.us

Nutrition Data

The Nutrition Data website includes links to a body mass index calculator, diet and exercise aids, a nutrition glossary, a recipe analysis program, and much, much more.
Website: www.nutritiondata.com

United States Department of Agriculture Food and Nutrition Service

The USDA's Food and Nutrition Service program provides children and low-income adults with access to food, a healthful diet, and nutrition education. Visit the website to see if you qualify for any of its programs.
Website: www.fns.usda.gov

ORGANIC FOODS AND HOUSEHOLD PRODUCTS

Food for Life Baking Company

Food for Life Baking Company offers all-natural baked goods, including breads, cereals, pastas, and more. Each line includes products developed to satisfy specific dietary requirements, such as wheat- and gluten-free, low-sodium, high-fiber, dairy-free, low-fat, and yeast-free. Browse the online catalogue or check the website for local retail outlets.
Website: www.foodforlife.com

Good Guide

This website's mission is to guide you in switching to non-toxic, environmentally healthy products. Healthy alternatives are suggested in several categories, including food, personal care items, and household cleaners.
Website: www.goodguide.com

Organic Valley Farms

Organic Valley Farms utilizes a cooperative business model and works through the efforts of numerous farmer-members all across the country. Click on the "Who's Your Farmer?" link to meet farmers near you and order their products.
Website: www.organicvalley.coop

References

Chapter 1

Barnett, E., Morley, P. "Diagnostic ultrasound in renal disease." *British Medical Bulletin*. Sep 1972; 28(3): 196–9.

Johnson, C.A., Levey, A.S. et al. "Clinical practice guidelines for chronic kidney disease in adults: Part II. Glomerular filtration rate, proteinuria, and other markers." *American Family Physician*. Sep 15, 2004; 70(6): 1091–7.

Murtagh, F.E., Addington-Hall, J.M. "Symptoms in advanced renal disease: A cross-sectional survey of system prevalence in stage 5 chronic kidney disease managed without dialysis." *Journal of Palliative Medicine*. Dec 2007; 10(6): 1266–76.

Chapter 2

Goransson, L.G. Bergrem, H. "Consequences of late referral of patients with end-stage renal disease." *Journal of Internal Medicine*. Aug 2001; 250(2): 154–9.

Johnson, C.A., Levey, A.S. et al. "Clinical practice guidelines for chronic kidney disease in adults: Part I. Definition, disease stages, evaluation, treatment, and risk factors." *American Family Physician*. Sep 1, 2004; 70(5): 869–76.

Lameire, N., Biesen, W.V., Vanholder, R. "Initiation of dialysis: Is the problem solved by NECOSAD?" *Nephrology Dialysis Transplantation*. Sep 2002; 17(9): 1550–2.

Malovrh, M. "Vascular access for hemodialysis: Arteriovenous fistula." *Therapeutic Apheresis and Dialysis*. Jun 2005; 9(3): 214–7.

Mange, K.C., Joffe, M.M., Feldman, H.I. "Dialysis prior to living donor kidney transplantation and rates of acute rejection." *Nephrology Dialysis Transplantation*. Jan 2003; 18(1): 172–7.

Mehrotra, R., Marsh, D. et al. "Patient education and access of ESRD patients to renal replacement therapies beyond in-center hemodialysis." *Kidney International*. Jul 2005; 68(1):378–90.

Neyhart, C.D. "Patient questions about transplantation: A resource guide." *Nephrology Nursing Journal.* May–Jun 2009; 36(3): 279–85.

Scandling, J.D. "Kidney transplant candidate evaluation." *Seminars in Dialysis.* Nov–Dec 2005; 18(6): 487–94.

Snyder, S., Pendergraph, P. "Detection and evaluation of chronic kidney disease." *American Family Physician.* Nov 1, 2005; 72(9): 1723–32.

Wood, C., Gonzalez, E.A., Martin, K.J. "Challenges in the therapy of secondary hyperparathyroidism." *Therapeutic Apheresis and Dialysis.* Feb 2005; 9(1):4–8.

Chapter 3

Barret, B.J. "Applying multiple interventions in chronic kidney disease." *Seminars in Dialysis.* Mar–Apr 2003; 16(2): 157–64.

Botton, W.K. "Nephrology nurse practitioners in a collaborative care model." *American Journal of Kidney Disease.* May 1998; 31(5): 786–93.

Rastogi, A., Linden, A., Nissenson, A.R. "Disease management in chronic kidney disease." *Advances in Chronic Kidney Disease.* Jan 2008; 15(1): 19–28.

Smith Jr., G.O. "The role of physician assistants in improving renal care." *Nephrology News and Issues.* Apr 2004; 18(5): 51–6.

Spry, L. "Building the chronic kidney disease management team." *Advances in Chronic Kidney Disease.* Jan 2008; 15(1): 29–36.

Chapter 4

Anway, M.D., Leathers, C. et al. "Endocrine disruptor vinclozolin induced epigenetic and transgenerational adult-onset disease." *Endocrinology.* Dec 2006; 147(12): 5515–23.

Cachofiero, V., Goicochea, M. et al. "Oxidative stress and inflammation: A link between chronic kidney disease and cardiovascular disease." *Kidney International.* 2008; 74: S4–S9.

Forbes, J.M., Fukami, K. et al. "Diabetic nephropathy: Where hemodynamics meets metabolism." *Experimental Clinics Endocrinology Diabetes.* Feb 2007;115(2): 69–84.

Pohlers, D., Brenmoehl, J. et al. "TGF-beta and fibrosis in different organs-molecular pathway imprints." *Biochimica et Biphysica Acta.* Aug 2009; 1792(8): 746–56.

Ronco, C., Chionh, C.Y. et al. "The cardiorenal syndrome." *Blood Purification.* 2009; 27(1): 114–26.

Schnaper, H.W., Jandeska, S. et al. "TGF-beta signal transduction in chronic kidney disease." *Frontiers in Bioscience.* Jan 1, 2009; 14:2448–65.

Solhaug, M.J., Bolger, P.M. et al. "The Developing Kidney and Environmental Toxins." *Pediatrics.* April 2004; 113 (4): 1084–91.

Valko, M., Morris, H. et al. "Metals, Toxicity, and Oxidative Stress." *Current Medicinal Chemistry.* May 2005; 12(10): 1161–1208.

Vaziri, N.D. "Causal Link Between Oxidative Stress, Inflammation, and Hypertension." *Iranian Journal of Kidney Diseases.* 2008; 2.

Chapter 5

Corpeleijn, E., Bakker, S.J., Stolk, R.P. "Obesity and impaired renal function: Potential for lifestyle intervention?" *European Journal of Epidemiology.* 2009; 24(6): 275–80.

Da Silva, A.A., Do Carmo, J., Dubinion, J., Hall, J.E. "The role of the sympathetic nervous system in obesity-related hypertension." *Current Hypertension Reports..* Jun 2009; 11(3): 206–11.

Dubel, G.J., Murphy, T.P. "The role of percutaneous revascularization for renal artery stenosis." *Vascular Medicine.* 2008; 13(2): 141–45.

Forbes, J.M., Fukami, K., Cooper, M.E. "Diabetic nephropathy: Where hemodynamics meets metabolism." *Experimental and Clinical Endocrinology and Diabetes.* Feb 2007; 115(2): 69–84.

Hall, J.E. "Pathophysiology of obesity hypertension." *Current Hypertension Reports.* Apr 2000; 2(2): 139–47.

Hou, F.F., Zhang, X. et al. "Efficacy and safety of benazepril for advanced chronic renal insufficiency." *The New England Journal of Medicine.* Jan 12, 2006; 354(2): 131–40.

Kawar, B., Bello, A.K., El Nahas, M. "High Prevalence of Microalbuminuria in the Overweight and Obese Population: Data from a UK Population Screening Programme." *Nephron Clinical Practice.* May 15, 2009; 112(3): c205–12.

Navaneethan, S.D., Nigwekar, S.U., Seghal, A.R., Strippoli, G.F. "Aldosterone antagonists for preventing the progression of chronic kidney disease: Systematic review and meta-analysis." *Clinical Journal of the American Society of Nephrology.* Mar 2009; 4(3): 542–51.

Navarro, J.F., Milena, F.J. et al. "Renal pro-inflammatory cytokine gene expression in diabetic nephropathy: Effect of angiotensin-converting enzyme inhibition and pentoxifylline administration." *American Journal of Nephrology.* 2006; 26(6): 562–70.

Ruggenenti, P., Bettinaglio, P., Pinares, F., Remuzzi, G. "Angiotensin converting enzyme insertion/deletion polymorphism and renoprotection in diabetic and non-diabetic nephropathies." *Clinical Journal of the American Society of Nephrology.* Sep 2008; 3(5): 1511–25.

Sanchez, A.P., Sharma, K. "Transcription factors in the pathogenesis of diabetic nephropathy." *Expert Reviews in Molecular Medicine.* April 28, 2009; 11: e13.

Savoia, C., Schiffrin, E.L. "Inflammation in Hypertension." *Current Opinion in Nephrology and Hypertension.* Mar 2006; 15(2): 152–8.

Textor, S.C. "Renovascular hypertension update." *Current Hypertension Reports.* Dec 2006; 8(6): 521–7.

Textor, S.C., Lerman, L., McKusick, M. "The uncertain value of renal artery interventions: Where are we now?" *JACC Cardiovascular Interventions.* Mar 2009; 2, 30: 175–82.

Thomson Reuters. *Physicians Desk Reference 2001.*

Thorn, L.M., Forsblom, C. et al. "Metabolic syndrome as a risk factor for cardiovascular disease, mortality, and progression of diabetic nephropathy in type 1 diabetes." *Diabetes Care.* May 2009; 32(5): 950–2.

Zelmanovitz, T., Gerchman, F., Balthazar, A.P. et al. "Diabetic nephropathy." *Diabetology & Metabolic Syndrome.* Sept 21, 2009; 1(1): 10.

Chapter 6

Appleton, N. *Stopping Inflammation: Relieving the Cause of Degenerative Diseases.* Garden City Park, NY: Square One Publishers, 2005.

Chang, M.Y., Ong, A.C. "Autosomal dominant polycystic kidney disease: Recent advances in pathogenesis and treatment." *Nephron Physiology.* 2008; 108(1): p1–7.

Demetriou, D., Tziakouri, C. et al. "Autosomal dominant polycystic kidney disease type 2: Ultrasound, genetic, and clinical correlations." *Nephrology Dialysis Transplantation.* 2000; 15(20): 205–11.

Ferri, C., Puccini, R. et al. "Low antigen-content diet in the treatment of patients with IgA Nephropathy." *Nephrology Dialysis Transplantation.* 1993; 8(11): 1193–8.

Hateboer, N., Van Dijk, M. et al. "Comparison of phenotypes of polycystic kidney disease types 1 and 2." *Lancet.* 1999; 353: 103–7.

Helma, C., Ubeis, F. "Celiac sprue-associated membranous nephropathy." *Clinical Nephrology.* Sep 2007; 68(3): 197.

Kodner, C. "Nephrotic syndrome in adults: Diagnosis and Management." *American Family Physician.* Nov 15, 2009; 80(10): 1129–34.

Lagrue, G., Laurent, J., Rostoker, G. "Food allergy and idiopathic nephritic syndrome." *Kidney International Supplement.* Nov 1989; 27: S147–51.

Laurent, J., Lagrue, G. "Dietary manipulation for idiopathic nephrotic syndrome: A new approach to therapy." *Allergy.* Nov 1989; 44(8): 599–603.

Laurent, J., Rostoker, G. et al. "Is adult idiopathic nephrotic syndrome food allergy? Value of oligoantigenic diets." *Nephron.* 1987;47(1): 7–11.

Ludvigsson, J.F., Mongtomery, S.M. et al. "Celiac disease and the risk of renal disease—a general population cohort study." *Nephrology Dialysis Transplantation.* Jul 2006; 21(7): 1809–15.

Sieniawska, M., Syzmanik-Grzelak, H. "The role of cow's milk protein intolerance in steroid-resistant nephrotic syndrome." *Acta Paediatrica.* Dec 1992; 81(12): 1007–12.

Chapter 7

Adhiyaman, V., Asghar, M. et al. "Nephrotoxicity in the elderly due to co-prescription of angiotensin converting enzyme inhibitors and nonsteroidal anti-inflammatory drugs." *Journal of the Royal Society of Medicine.* Oct 2001; 94(10): 512–4.

Al Shohaib, S., Raweily, E. "Acute tubular necrosis due to captopril." *American Journal of Nephrology.* Mar-Apr 2000; 20(2): 149–152.

Barri, Y.M., Munshi, N.C. et al. "Podocyte injury associated glomerulopathies induced by pamidronate." *Kidney International.* Feb 2004; 65(2): 634–41.

Cheung, C.M., Ponnusamy, A., Anderton, J.G. "Management of acute renal failure in the elderly patient: A clinician's guide." *Drugs Aging.* 2008; 25(6): 455–76.

Delmas, P.D. "Non-steroidal inflammatory drugs and renal function." *British Journal of Rheumatology.* Apr 1995; 34 Suppl 1: 25–8.

Diel, I.J., Bergner, R., Grotz, K.A. "Adverse effects of bisphosphonates: Current issues." *Journal of Supportive Oncology.* Nov-Dec 2007; 475–82.

Guru, V., Fremes, S.E. "The role of N-acetylcysteine in preventing radiographic contrast—induced nephropathy." *Clinical Nephrology.* Aug 2004; 62(2): 77–83.

Halimi, J.M., Asmar, R., Ribstein, J. "Optimal nephrotection: Use, misuse, and misconceptions about blockade of the renin-angiotensin system. Lessons from the ON TARGET and other recent trials." *Diabetes and Metabolism.* Dec 2009; 36(6): 455–76.

John, R., Herxenberg, A.M. "Renal toxicity of therapeutic drugs." *Journal of Clinical Pathology.* Jun 2009; 62(6): 505–515.

Kleinknecht, D., Kanfer, A., Morel-Maroger, L., Mery, J.P. "Immunologically mediated drug-induced renal failure." *Contributions to Nephrology.* 1978; 10: 42–52.

Krishnamurthy, M., Snyder, R., Bachurina, M. "Long-term use of proton pump inhibitors: Are they really safe? A case of delayed acute interstitial nephritis." *Journal of the American Geriatrics Society.* Aug 2009; 57(8): 1513–4.

Mandal, A.K., Matkert, R.J. "Diuretics potentiate angiotensin converting enzyme-inhibitor acute renal failure." *Clinical Nephrology.* Sep 1994; 42(3): 170–4.

Markowitz, G.S., Stokes, M.B., Radhakrishnan, J., D'Agati, V.D. "Acute phosphate nephropathy following oral sodium phosphate bowel purgative: An underrecognized cause of chronic renal failure." *Journal of the American Society of Nephrology.* Nov 2005; 16(11): 3398–96.

Mueller, C. "Prevention of contrast-induced nephropathy with volume supplementation." *Kidney International Supplement.* Apr 2006; S16–9.

Mueller-Lenke, N., Buerkle, G. et al. "Incidence of contrast-induced nephropathy with volume supplementation: Insights from a large cohort." *Medical Principles and Practice.* 2008; 17(5): 409–14.

Parra, D., Legreid, A.M., Beckey, N.P., Reyes, S. "Metformin monitoring and change in serum creatinine levels in patients undergoing radiologic procedures involving administration of intravenous contrast media." *Pharmacotherapy.* Aug 2004; 24(8): 987–93.

Radford, M.G., Holley, K.E. et al. "Reversible membranous nephropathy associated with the use of non-steroidal anti-inflammatory drugs." *JAMA.* Aug 14, 1996; 276(6): 466–9.

Schlaudecker, J.D., Bernheisel, C.R. "Gadolinium-associated nephrogenic systemic fibrosis." *American Family Physician.* Oct 1, 2009; 80(7): 711–4.

Chapter 8

Anderson, J., Glynn, L.G. "The impact of renal insufficiency and anemia on survival in patients with cardiovascular disease: A cohort study." *BMC Cardiovascular Disorders.* Nov 12, 2009; 9: 51.

Andress, D.L., Coyne, D.W. "Management of secondary hyperparathyroidism in stages 3 and 4 chronic kidney disease." *Endocrine Practice.* Jan–Feb 2008; 14(1): 18–27.

Cachofiero, V., Goichochea, M. et al. "Oxidative stress and inflammation: A link between chronic kidney disease and cardiovascular disease." *Kidney International.* Dec 2008; 74: S4–S9.

Goldberg, A., Hammerman, H. "Inhospital and 1-year mortality of patients who develop worsening renal function following acute ST-elevation myocardial infarction." *American Heart Journal.* Aug 2005; 150(2): 330–7.

Hadland, B.K., Longmore, G.D. "Erythroid-stimulating agents in cancer therapy: potential dangers and biologic mechanisms." *Journal of Clinical Oncology.* Sep 1, 2009; 27(25): 4217–26.

Kalantar-Zadeh, K., Mehrotra, R., Fouque, D., Kopple, J.D. "Metabolic acidosis and malnutrition—inflammation complex in chronic renal failure." *Seminars in Dialysis.* Nov–Dec 2004; 17(6): 455–65.

Kopple, J.D., Kalantar-Zadeh, K., Mehrotra, R. "Risks of chronic metabolic acidosis in patients with chronic kidney disease." *Kidney International Supplement.* Jun 2005; (95): S21–7.

Mathur, R.P., Dash, S.C. "Effects of correction of metabolic acidosis on blood urea and bone metabolism in patients with mild to moderate kidney disease: A prospective randomized single blind controlled trial." *Renal Failure.* 2006; 28(1): 1–5.

Rosen-Zvi, B., Gafter-Gvili, A. et al. "Intravenous versus oral iron supplementation for the treatment of anemia in CKD: Systematic review and meta-analysis." *American Journal of Kidney Disease.* Nov 2008; 52(5): 897–906.

Saliba, W., El-Haddad, B. "Secondary hyperparathyroidism: Pathophysiology and treatment." *Journal of the American Board of Family Medicine.* Sep–Oct 2009; 22(5): 574–81.

Schiffrin, E.L., Lipman, M.L., Mann, J.F. "Chronic kidney disease: Effects on the cardiovascular system." *Circulation.* July 3, 2007; 116(1): 85–97.

Singh, A.K., Sczcech, L. et al. "Correction of anemia with epoietin alfa in kidney disease." *New England Journal of Medicine.* Nov 16, 2006; 355(20): 2085–98.

Chapter 9

Barretta, R. "A Summary of the Results of a 14 Week Deep Exercise Program on Selected Components of Fitness." *Journal of Aquatic Physical Therapy.* 1995; 3(3): 19–25.

Ettinger, W.H., Burns, R. et al. "A randomized trial comparing aerobic exercise and resistance exercise with a health education program in older patients with osteoarthritis." *JAMA.* Jan 1,1997; 277(1): 25–31.

Fored, C.M., Ejerblad, E. et al. "Acetaminophen, aspirin and chronic renal failure." *New England Journal of Medicine.* Dec 2001; 345(25): 1801–08.

Garg, A.X., Moist, L. et al. "Risk of hypertension and reduced kidney function after acute gastroenteritis from bacteria-contaminated drinking water." *Canadian Association Medical Journal.* Aug 2, 2005; 173(3): 261–8.

Iseki, K., Tohyama, K., Matsumoto, T., Nakamyra, H. "High prevalence of kidney disease among patients with sleep related breathing disorder." *Hypertension Research.* Feb 2008; 31(2): 249–55.

Jarup, L. "Land contamination and renal dysfunction." *Occupational and Environmental Medicine.* 2003: 60: 451–462.

Kuehn, B.M., "Traces of Drugs Found in Drinking Water." *JAMA.* 2008; 299(17): 2011–13.

Lyon, C.C., Turney, J.H. "Pseudoephedrine toxicity in renal failure." *British Journal of Clinical Practice.* Oct-Nov 1996; 50(70): 396–7.

Markell, M.S. "Potential benefit of complementary medicine modalities in patients with chronic kidney disease." *Advances in Chronic Kidney Disease.* Jul 2005; 12(3): 292–9.

Moist, L.M., Sentrop, J.M. et al. "Risk of pregnancy-related hypertension within five years of exposure to bacteria-contaminated drinking water." *Kidney International Supplement.* Feb 2009; (112): S47–9.

Muntner, P., He, J. et al. "Blood lead and chronic kidney disease in the general United States population: Results from NHANES III." *Kidney International.* 2003; 63: 1040–50.

Murray, M.D., Brater, D.C. "Effects of NSAIDS on the kidney." *Progress in Drug Research.* 1997; 49: 155–71.

Navas-Acien, A., Tellez-Plaza, M. et al. "Blood cadmium and lead and chronic kidney disease in US adults." *American Journal of Epidemiology.* Nov 1, 2009; 170(9): 1156–64.

Orth, S.R., Hallan, S.I. "Smoking: A risk factor for progression of chronic kidney disease and for cardiovascular morbidity and mortality in some patients—absence of evidence or evidence of absence?" *Clinical Journal of the American Society of Nephrology.* Jan 2008; (1): 226–36.

Salerno, S.M., Jackson, J.L., Berbano, E.P. "Effect of oral pseudoephedrine on blood pressure and heart rate: A meta-analysis." *Archives of Internal Medicine.* Aug 8-22, 2005; 165(15): 1686–94.

Sobh, M.A. "Environmental Pollution Is Increasing the Incidence of Chronic Renal Failure." *Toxin Reviews.* 1996; 15(3): 199–205.

Taylor-Piliae, R.E. "Tai chi as an adjunct to cardiac rehabilitation exercise training." *Journal of Cardiopulmonary Rehabilitation and Prevention.* Mar–Apr 2003; 23(2): 90–6.

Thorsteinsdottir, B., Grande, J.P., Garovic, V.D. "Acute renal failure in a young weight lifter taking multiple food supplements, including creatine monohydrate." *Journal of Renal Nutrition.* Oct 2006; 16(4):341–5.

Walton, K.G., Pugh, N.D., Gelderloos, P., Macrae, P. "Stress reduction and preventing hypertension: Preliminary support for a psychoneuroendocrine mechanism." *Journal of Alternative and Complementary Medicine.* Fall 1995; (3): 263–83.

Wedeen, R.P. "Occupational and environmental renal disease." *Seminars in Nephrology.* Jan 1997; 17(1): 46–53.

Whelton, A., Hamilton, C.W. "Nonsteroidal anti-inflammatory drugs: Effects on kidney function." *Journal of Clinical Pharmacology.* Jul 1991; 31(7): 588–98.

Wolk, R., Shamsuzzaman, A.S., Somers, V.K. "Obesity, sleep apnea and hypertension." *Hypertension.* Dec 2003; 42(6): 1067–74.

Chapter 10

Abol-Enein, H., Gheith, O.A. et al. "Ionized alkaline water: New strategy for the treatment of metabolic acidosis in experimental animals." *Therapeutic Apheresis and Dialysis..* Jun 2009; 13(3): 220–4.

Appleton, N. *Stopping Inflammation: Relieving the Cause of Degenerative Diseases.* Garden City Park, NY: Square One Publishers, 2005.

Coppo, R., Amore, A., Roccatello, D. "Dietary antigens and primary immunoglobulin A nephropathy." *Journal of the American Society of Nephrology.* Apr 1992; 2(10 Suppl): S173–80.

Coppo, R., Basolo, B. et al. "Mediterranean diet and primary IgA nephropathy." *Clinical Nephrology.* Aug 1986; 26(2): 72–82.

Ferri, C., Puccini, R. et al. "Low antigen-content diet in the treatment of patients with IgA nephropathy." *Nephrology Dialysis Transplantation.* 1993; 8(11): 1193–8.

He, F.J., MacGregor, G.A. "Effect of modest salt reduction on blood pressure: A meta-analysis of randomized trials. Implications for public health." *Journal of Human Hypertension.* Nov 2002; 16(11): 761–70.

Kirkken, J.A., Laverman, G.D., Navis, G. "Benefits of dietary sodium restriction in the management of chronic kidney disease." *Current Opinion in Nephrology and Hypertension.* Nov 2009; 18(6): 531–8.

Levitan, E.B., Wolk, A., Mittleman, M.A. "Consistency with the DASH diet and incidence of heart failure." *Archives of Internal Medicine.* May 11, 2009; 169(9): 851–7.

Ludvigsson, J.F., Mongtomery, S.M. et al. "Celiac disease and the risk of renal disease: A general population cohort study." *Nephrology Dialysis Transplantation.* Jul 2006; 21(7): 1809-15.

Menon, V., Kopple, J.D., Wang, X. et al. "Effect of a very low protein diet on outcomes: Long term follow-up of the Modification of Diet in Renal Disease (MDRD) study." *American Journal of Kidney Diseases.* Feb 2009; 53(2): 208–17.

Pennington, Jean A.T., Spungen, Judith. *Bowes and Church's Food Values of Portions Commonly Used, 19th Edition.* Philadelphia: Lippincott Williams & Wilkins, 2010.

Rozinn, A.P., Lewin, M. et al. "Essential mixed cryoglobulinemia type II." *Clinical and Experimental Rheumatology.* May–Jun 2006; 24(3): 329–32.

Toto, R.D. "Treatment of hypertension in chronic kidney disease." *Seminars in Nephrology.* Nov 2005; 25(6): 435–9.

Walser, M., Hill, S. "Can renal replacement be deferred by a supplemented very low protein diet?" *Journal of the American Society of Nephrology.* Jan 1999; 10(1): 110–6.

Young, R.O., Young, S.R. *The pH Miracle: Balance Your Diet, Reclaim Your Health.* New York: Wellness Central, 2002.

Calorie Count: www.caloriecount.com

The Daily Plate: www.thedailyplate.com

Food for Life: www.foodforlife.com

Nephron Information Center: www.foodvalues.us

Chapter 11

An, W., Kim, H.J., Cho, K.H., Vaziri, N.D. "Omega-3 fatty acid supplementation attenuates oxidative stress, inflammation, and tubulointerstitial fibrosis in the remnant kidney." *American Journal of Physiology Renal Physiology.* Oct 2009; 297(4): F895–903.

Babaei-Jadidi, R., Karachalias, N., Ahmed, N. et al. "Prevention of incipient diabetic nephropathy by high-dose thiamine and benfotiamine." *Diabetes.* Aug 2003; 52 (8): 2110–20.

Blair, D. "Vitamin supplementation and CKD." *Renal & Urology News.* June 15, 2009.

Bordelon, P., Ghetu, M.V., Langan, R.C. "Recognition and management of vitamin D deficiency." *American Family Physician.* Oct 15, 2009; 80 (8): 841–6.

Chan, W., Krieg, R.J., Norkus, E.P., Chan, J.C. "Alpha-Tocopherol reduces proteinuria, oxidative stress, and expression of transforming growth factor beta 1 in IgA nephropathy in the rat." *Molecular Genetics and Metabolism.* Mar 1998; 63(3): 224–9.

Dhonukshe-Rutten, R.A., Pluijm, S.A., de Groot, L.C. et al. "Homocysteine and vitamin B12 status relate to bone turnover markers, broadband ultrasound attenuation, and fractures in healthy elderly people." *Journal of Bone and Mineral Research.* Jun 2005; 20 (6): 921–9.

Kuhad, A., Chopra, K. "Attenuation of diabetic nephropathy by tocotrienol: Involvement of NFkB signaling pathway." *Life Sciences.* Feb 27, 2009; 84(9-10): 296–301.

Kuhad, A., Tirkey, N., Pilkhwal, S., Chopra, K. "Effects of spirulina, a blue green algae on gentamicin-induced oxidative stress and renal dysfunction in rats." *Fundamental and Clinical Pharmacology.* Apr 2006; 20(2): 121–28.

Lauretani, F., Maggio, M., Pizzarelli F. et al. "Omega-3 and renal function in older adults." *Current Pharmaceutical Design.* 2009; 15(36):4149–56.

Lee, S.J., Kang, J.G. et al. "Effects of alpha-lipoic acid on transforming growth factor beta 1-p38 mitogen-activated protein kinase-fibronectin pathway in diabetic nephropathy." *Metabolism.* May 2009; 58, 50:616–23.

Lee, W.H., Akatsuka, S., Shirase, T. et al. "Alpha-tocopherol induces calnexin in renal tubular cells: Another protective mechanism against free radical-induced cellular damage." *Archives of Biochemistry and Biophysics.* Sep 15, 2006; 453(2): 168–78,

Littarru, G.P., Tiano, L. "Bioenergetic and antioxidant properties of coenzyme Q10: recent developments." *Molecular Biotechnology.* Sep 2007; 37(1): 31–7.

Looker, A.C., Pfeiffer, C.M. et al. "Serum 25 hydroxyvitamin status of the US population: 1988–1994 compared with 2000–2004." *The American Journal of Clinical Nutrition.* 2008 Dec; 88(6): 1519–27.

McHugh, G.J., Graber, M.L., Freebaiurn, R.C. "Fatal vitamin C-associated renal failure." *Anesthesia and intensive care.* Jul 2008; 36(4): 585–8.

McLean, B.B., Jacques, P.F., Selhub et al. "Plasma B vitamins, homocysteine, and their relation with bone loss and hip fracture in elderly men and women." *Journal of Clinical Endocrinology and Metabolism.* Jun 2008; 93(6): 2206–12.

Porrini, M., Simonetti, P., Ciappellano, S. et al. "Thiamine, riboflavin, and pyridoxine status in chronic renal insufficiency." *International Journal of Vitamin and Nutrition Research.* 1989; 59(3): 304–88.

Rabbani, N., Alam, S.S., Riaz, S. et al. "High-dose thiamine therapy for patients with type 2 diabetes and microalbuminuria: A randomized, double-blind placebo-controlled pilot study." *Diabetologia.* Feb 2009; 52 (2): 208–12.

Samuels, R., Mani, U.V., Iyer, U.M., Nayak, U.S. "Hypocholeterolemic effect of spirulina in patients with hyperlipidemic nephrotic syndrome." *Journal of Medicinal Food.* Summer 2002; 5(2): 91–6.

Shea, M.K., Booth, S.L. "Update on the role of vitamin K in skeletal health." *Nutrition Review.* Oct 2008; 66(10): 549–57.

Torres-Duran, P.V., Ferreira-Hermosillo, A., Juarez-Oropeza, M.A. "Antihyperlipemic and antihypertensive effects of *Spirulina maxima* in an open sample of Mexican population: A preliminary report." *Lipids in Health and Disease.* Nov 26, 2007; 6:33.

Trachtman, H. et al. "Vitamin E ameliorates renal injury in an experimental model of IgA nephropathy." *Pediatric Research.* Oct 1996; 40(4): 620–6.

Upaganlawar, A., Farswan, M., Rathod, S., Balaraman, R. "Modification of biochemical parameters of gentamicin nephrotoxicity and green tea in rats." *Indian Journal of Experimental Biology.* May 2006; 44(5): 416–8.

Chapter 12

Ahmed, M.S., Hou, S.H. et al. "Treatment of idiopathic membranous nephropathy with the herb *Astragalus membranaceus.*" *American Journal of Kidney Disease.* Dec 2007; 50 (6): 1028–32.

Aviram, M., Dornfeld, L. "Pomegranate juice consumption inhibits serum angiotensin converting enzyme activity and reduces systolic blood pressure." *Atherosclerosis.* Sep 2001; 158(1): 195–8.

Banerjee, S.K., Mukherjee, P.K., Maulik, S.K. "Garlic as an antioxidant: The good, the bad, the ugly." *Phytotherapy Research.* Feb 2003; 17(2): 97–106.

Bardana Jr, E.J., Malinow, M.R. et al. "Diet induced systemic lupus erythematosus in primates." *American Journal of Kidney Diseases.* May 1982; 1(6): 345–52.

Basu, A., Penoganda, K. "Pomegranate juice: A heart healthy fruit juice." *Nutrition Reviews.* Jan 2009; 67(1): 49–56.

Chen, L.P., Zhou, Q.L., Yang, J.H. "Protective effects of astragali injection on tubular in patients with primary nephrotic syndrome." *Journal of Central South University Medical Sciences.* Apr 2004; 29(2): 152–3.

Clare, B.A., Conroy, R.S., Spelman, K. "The diuretic effect in human subjects of an extract of *Taraxacum officinale folium* over a single day." *Journal of Alternative and Complementary Medicine.* Aug 15, 2009; 15(8): 929–34.

Drobiova, H., Thomson, M. "Garlic increases antioxidant levels in diabetic and hypertensive rats determined by a modified peroxidase method." *Evidence-Based Complementary and Alternative Medicine.* Feb 20, 2009.

Duke, J.A. *The Green Pharmacy Herbal Handbook.* Emmaus, PA: Rodale Press, 2000.

Fetrow, C.W., Avila, J.R. *The Complete Guide to Herbal Medicines.* New York: Pocket Books, 2000.

Flanagan, R.J., Meredith, T.J. "Use of N-acetylcysteine in clinical toxicology." *The American Journal of Medicine.* Sep 30, 1991; 91(3C): 131S–39S.

Friedman, E. "Can the bowel substitute for the kidney in advanced renal failure?" *Current Medical Research and Opinion.* Aug 2009; 25(8): 1913–8.

Gedeke, J., Noble, N.A., Border, W.A. "Curcumin blocks multiple sites of the TGF-beta signaling cascade in renal cells." *Kidney International.* Jul 2004; 66(1): 112–120.

Jutte, R., Riley, D. "A review of the use and role of low potencies in homeopathy." *Complementary Therapies in Medicine.* Dec 2005; 13(4): 291–6.

Kaur, G., Athar, M., Alam, M.S. "Dietary supplementation of silymarin protects against chemically induced nephrotoxicity, inflammation, and renal tumor promotion response." *Investigational New Drugs.* Jul 10, 2009.

Kim, H.Y., Kang, K.S. et al. "Protective effect of heat processed American ginseng against diabetic renal damage in rats." *Journal of Agricultural and Food Chemistry.* Oct 17, 2007; 55(21): 8491–7.

Kim, H.Y., Kang, K.S., Yamabe, N., Yokozawa, T. "Comparison of the effects of Korean ginseng and heat-processed Korean ginseng on diabetic oxidative stress." *The American Journal of Chinese Medicine.* 2008; 36(5): 989–1004.

Lin, J.L. et al. "Long-term outcome of repeated lead chelation therapy in progressive non-diabetic chronic kidney diseases." *Nephrology Dialysis Transplantation.* Oct 2007; 22(10): 2924–31.

Lin, J.L., Lin-Tan, D.T. et al. "Low-level environmental exposure to lead and progressive chronic kidney disease." *American Journal of Medicine.* Aug 2006; 119(8): 707.e1–9.

Luyckx, V.A., Ballantine, R. et al. "Herbal remedy associated acute renal failure secondary to Cape aloes." *American Journal of Kidney Disease.* Mar 2002; 39(3): E 13.

Lynch, D.M. "Cranberry for Prevention of Urinary Tract Infections." *American Family Physician.* 2004; 70: 2175–77.

Malinow, M.R. et al. "Systemic lupus erythematosus-like syndrome in monkeys fed alfalfa sprouts: Role of a nonprotein amino acid." *Science.* Apr 23, 1982; 216(4544): 415–17.

Murugavel, P., Pari, L. et al. "Cadmium induced mitochondrial injury and apoptosis in vero cells: Protective effect of diallyl tetrasulfide from garlic." *International Journal of Biochemistry and Cell Biology.* 2007; 39(1): 161–70.

Ranganathan, N., Friedman, E. et al. "Probiotic dietary supplementation in patients with stage 3 and 4 chronic kidney disease: A 6-month pilot scale trial in Canada." *Current Medical Research and Opinion.* Aug 2009; 25(8): 1919–30.

Ribaldo, P.D., Souza, D.S. et al. "Green tea (*Camellia sinensis*) attenuates nephropathy by downregulating Nox4 NADPH oxidase in diabetic spontaneously hypertensive rats." *Journal of Nutrition.* Jan 2009; 139(1): 96–100.

Rigelsky, J.M., Sweet, B.V. "Hawthorn: Pharmacology and therapeutic uses." *American Journal of Health-System Pharmacy.* Mar 1, 2002; 59(5): 417–22.

Salamon, E., Zhu, W., Stefano, G.B. "Nitric oxide as a possible mechanism for understanding the therapeutic effects of osteopathic manipulative medicine (Review)." *International Journal of Molecular Medicine.* Sep 2004; 14(3): 443–9.

Senapati, S.K., Dey, S., Dwivedi, S.K., Swarup, D. "Effect of garlic (*Allium sativum L.*) extract on tissue lead level in rats." *Journal of Ethnopharmacology.* Aug 2001; 76(3): 229–32.

Sharma, S., Kulkarni, S.K., Chopra, K. "Curcumsin, the active principle of turmeric (*Curcuma longa*) ameliorates diabetic nephropathy in rats." *Clinical and Experimental Pharmacology and Physiology.* Oct 2006; 33(10): 940–5.

Spiegel, A.J., Capobianco, J.D., Kruger, A., Spinner, W.D. "Osteopathic manipulative medicine in the treatment of hypertension: An alternative, conventional approach." *Heart Disease.* Jul-Aug 2003; 5(4): 272–8.

Su, L., Mao, J.C., Gu, J.H. "Effect of intravenous drip infusion of cyclophosphamide with high-dose Astragalus injection in treating lupus nephritis." *Journal of Chinese Integrative Medicine.* May 2007; 5(3): 272–5.

Trivedi, H., Daram, S. et al. "High-dose N-acetylcysteine for the prevention of contrast-induced nephropathy." *The American Journal of Medicine.* Sep 2009; 122(9): 874.e9–e.15.

Vasoo, S. "Drug induced lupus: An update." *Lupus.* 2006; 15(11): 757–761.

Zhang, Y.W., Wu, C.Y., Cheng, J.T. "Merit of Astragalus polysaccharide in the improvement of early diabetic nephropathy with an effect on mRNA expression of NF-kappaB and lkappa B in renal cortex of streptozotoxin-induced diabetic rats." *Journal of Ethnopharmacology.* Dec 3, 2007; 114(3): 387–92.

Zijlstra, F.J., van den Berg-De Lange, I., Huygen, F.J., Klein, J. "Anti-inflammatory actions of acupuncture." *Mediators of Inflammation.* Apr 2003; 12(2): 59–69.

Natural Medicines Comprehensive Database: www.naturaldatabase.com

Chapter 13

Cousins, Norman. *Anatomy of an Illness as Perceived by the Patient.* New York: W.W. Norton and Company, 2005.

Hassed, C. "How humour keeps you well." *Australian Family Physician.* Jan 2001; 30(1): 25–8.

Olshansky, B., Dossey, L. "Retroactive prayer: A preposterous hypothesis?" *British Medical Journal.* Dec 20, 2003; 327(7429): 1465–8.

Palmer, R.F., Katerndahl, D., Morgan-Kidd, J. "A randomized trial of the effects of remote intercessory prayer. Interactions with personal beliefs on problem-specific outcomes and functional status." *Journal of Complementary and Alternative Medicine.* Jun 2004; 10(3): 438–48.

Pothulaki, M., Macdonald, R.A. et al. "An investigation of the effects of music on anxiety and pain perception in patients undergoing hemodialysis treatment." *Journal of Health Psychology.* Oct 2008; 13(7): 912–20.

$\mathcal{I}$ndex

A

ACE and ACE inhibitors. *See* Angiotensin converting enzyme.

Acetaminophen. *See* Medications and tests, negative side effects of.

Acid-alkaline balance. *See* Diet, effects of, on kidney health; pH balance.

Acidosis. *See* pH balance.

Acupuncture. *See* Complementary therapies.

Adrenal gland, 8

ALA supplements. *See* Supplements, effects of.

Albumin, 21, 46

Albuminuria, 21

Allergens, 40

Alpha blockers, 56

Alpha lipoic acid (ALA) supplements. *See* Supplements, effects of.

Alternative therapies. *See* Complementary therapies.

Anemia, 22, 85
treatment of, 86

Angiodema, 49

Angiogram, 62

Angioplasty, 62, 81

Angiotensin converting enzyme (ACE), 47
inhibitors, 42, 48–49, 53–54, 71, 77–78

Angiotensin receptor blockers (ARBs), 42, 48–49, 53, 78

Antibiotics. *See* Medications and tests, negative side effects of.

ARBs. *See* Angiotensin receptor blockers.

Atherosclerosis, 41, 46, 51, 59
diagnosis of, 61
symptoms of, 60
treatment of, 61–63

Atkins diet. *See* Diet, effects of, on kidney health.

B

Benign prostatic hyperplasia (BPH), 72

Beta blockers, 55–56

Bicarbonate. *See* pH balance.

Bisphosphonates. *See* Medications and tests, negative side effects of.

Blood in urine. *See* Hematuria.
Blood pressure
  reading your, at home, 98–99
  regulation of, 7–8
  See also Hypertension; Renin-
    angiotensin-aldosterone system.
Blood sugar
  and kidney disease, 47–48,
  monitoring, 98–99
Blood tests
  blood urea nitrogen (BUN), 15
  creatinine, 14
  electronic GFR (eGFR), 13, 22
  glomerular filtration rate
    (GFR), 13, 19–20
Blood urea nitrogen (BUN). *See* Blood
  tests.
Body-building supplements. *See*
  Supplements, effects of.
BPH. *See* Benign prostatic hyperplasia.
BUN. *See* Blood tests.

C

Caffeine. *See* Medications and
  tests, negative side effects of.
Calcium supplements. *See*
  Supplements, effects of.
Calcium channel blockers, 53–54
Cardiac catheterization dye. *See*
  Medications and tests,
  negative side effects of.
Cardio-renal syndrome, 41
Case manager, 29, 31
CAT scan. *See* Medications and
  tests, negative side effects of;
  Tests of kidney function.
Chelation. *See* Complementary
  therapies.
Chiropractic medicine. *See*
  Complementary therapies.
Cholesterol, reducing, 50
Chronic kidney disease, definition of, 9

CKD. *See* Chronic kidney disease.
Clinics for the treatment of chronic
  kidney disease. *See* Kidney disease.
Coenzyme Q_{10} supplements.
  See Supplements, effects of.
Colonoscopy. *See* Medications and
  tests, negative side effects of.
Complementary health providers, 30
Complementary therapies
  acupuncture, 147
  chelation, 147
  chiropractic medicine, 146
  homeopathy, 147
  massage, 30, 146
  meditation, 148
  osteopathy, 146
  spiritual and emotional, 149–155
Creatinine. *See* Blood tests.
Cytokines, 38–39, 47

D

DASH diet. *See* Diet, effects of,
  on kidney health; Hyper-tension,
  treatment of.
Diabetic nephropathy, 46–47
  treatment of, 47–50
Dialysis, 23–25
  hemodialysis (HD), 24
  peritoneal (PD), 25
Diet, effects of, on kidney health
  acid-alkaline, 114, 116–118, 122
  Atkins, 116
DASH, 114
  fluid restriction, 107
  juicing, 118
  low-glycemic, 115
  magnesium, 113
  phosphorus, 87, 102, 112, 114
  potassium, 108–110
  protein, 110–112
  sodium, 106–108

Dietary alternatives, examples of
  at breakfast, 119–120
  at dinner, 121–122
  at lunch, 120–121
Diuretics, 54–55, 79
Dizziness. *See* Anemia.
Doctor's office visit
  checklist for, 32–33
  preparing for, 32

E

Edema, 12, 54, 66–67
  treatment of, 69, 79, 104,
    106, 108, 141–142, 146
eGFR. *See* Electronic GFR
Electrolytes, 7
Electronic GFR (eGFR), 13, 22
Endocrinologist, 30
Environmental toxins, 40–41,
    95, 104, 113, 143–147
Erythropoietin, 8, 22, 85
Exercise and weight loss. *See* Kidney
    health, improvement of.

F

Fibrosis, 39, 47, 52. *See also*
    Nephrogenic systemic fibrosis.
Fistula, 24
Fluid restriction. *See* Diet, effects
    of, on kidney health.
Free radicals, 38–39

G

Gadolinium. *See* Medications and
    tests, negative side effects of.
GFR. *See* Glomerular filtration rate.
Glomerular filtration rate (GFR),
    13, 19–20
Glomeruli, 6–7, 66. *See also*
    Glomerular filtration rate.
Glomerulonephritis (GN), 39, 65–66

  treatment of, 69
GN. *See* Glomerulonephritis.
Goodpasture's syndrome, 67

H

HD. *See* Dialysis.
Healthcare providers, 27–31
Hematuria, 11, 66
  signs of, 11
Hemoglobin, 22, 85
Herbal supplements. *See*
    Supplements, effects of.
Hgb. *See* Hemoglobin.
High blood pressure. *See*
    Hypertension.
Homeopathy. *See* Complementary
    therapies.
Homocysteine, 60, 126–127
Hypertension
  diagnosis of, 51, 98
  effects of, on kidneys, 51
  stages of, 52
  treatment of, 52–57, 114–115

I

Incontinence, 12
Inflammation
  causes of, 35–41, 46, 68–69
  effects of, 41
  high-level syndromes of, 65
  medications for, 42
  preventing, 42
Interstitial nephritis, 75
Itching. *See* Uremic symptoms.

J

Juicing. *See* Diet, effects of,
    on kidney health.

K

KEEP. *See* Kidney Early
   Evaluation Program.
Kidney disease
   acute, 9
   causes of, 8–9, 35, 45–63
   chronic (CKD), 9
   clinics for the treatment
      of chronic, 31
   polycystic, 9, 36, 65, 70–71
   stages of, 19–26
   symptoms of, 10–13, 20
Kidney Early Evaluation
   Program (KEEP), 16
Kidney function tests. *See*
   Tests of kidney function.
Kidney health, improvement of
   through exercise and weight loss,
      93–95
   through sleep, 96–97
   through quitting smoking, 95
   through stress reduction, 95
Kidneys
   function of, 6–8, 87
   location of, 5

L

Loss of appetite. *See* Uremic symptoms.
Low-glycemic diet. *See* Diet,
   effects of, on kidney health.
Lupus, 65–66

M

Magnesium. *See* Diet, effects
   of, on kidney health;
   Supplements, effects of.
Magnetic Resonance Imaging. *See*
   Medications and tests, negative
   side effects of, gadolinium; Tests
   of kidney function.

Massage. *See* Complementary
   therapies.
Medications and tests, negative
   side effects of
   acetatminophen, 100
   antibiotics, 76
   bisphophonates, 77
   caffeine, 101
   cardiac catheterization dye, 81
   CAT scan dye, 73, 80
   colonoscopy, 79
   gadolinium, 80, 82–83
   non-steroidal anti-inflammatory
      drugs (NSAIDs), 76, 79, 100
   phosphorus, 79
   proton-pump inhibitors (PPI), 76
   pseudoephedrine, 101
Meditation. *See* Complementary
   therapies.
Metallic taste. *See* Uremic symptoms.
MRI. *See* Medications and tests,
   negative side effects of,
   gadolinium; Tests of kidney
   function.

N

Nausea. *See* Uremic symptoms.
Nephritis, 11. *See also*
   Glomerulonephritis; Hematuria;
   Interstitial nephritis.
Nephrogenic systemic fibrosis, 83
Nephrologist, 13, 23, 28
Nephropathy, 46–47
   acute phosphate, 79
Nephrotic syndrome, 39–40, 65
   diagnosis of, 67–68
   treatment of, 69
Nocturia, 11
Non-steroidal anti-inflammatory
   drugs (NSAIDs). *See* Medications
   and tests, negative side effects of.

NP. *See* Nurse practitioner.
NSAIDs. *See* Medications and tests, negative side effects of.
Nurse practitioner (NP), 29
Nutritionist, 28–29, 31

O

Obesity
and hypertension, 57–58
and kidney disease, 57–59
and metabolic syndrome, 58
and proteinuria, 58
Office visit. *See* Doctor's office visit.
Omega-3 fatty acid supplements. *See* Supplements, effects of.
Osteopathy. *See* Complementary therapies.
Oxidative stress, 38–39

P

PA. *See* Physician assistants.
PAD. *See* Peripheral arterial disease.
Parathyroid hormone, 22, 86
PD. *See* Dialysis.
Peripheral arterial disease (PAD), 41, 59
pH balance
and acidosis, 87–88, 114, 116–118, 122
role of bicarbonate in, 7, 88, 117
Phosphorus. *See* Diet, effects of, on kidney health; Medications and tests, negative side effects of.
Physician assistants (PA), 29–30
Physician's office visit. *See* Doctor's office visit.
Polycystic kidney disease. *See* Kidney disease.
Potassium. *See* Diet, effects of, on kidney health; Supplements, effects of.

PPI. *See* Medications and tests, negative side effects of.
Primary care doctor, 28
Probiotic supplements. *See* Supplements, effects of.
Protein. *See* Diet, effects of, on kidney health.
Protein in urine. *See* Proteinuria.
Proteinuria, 11, 15–16, 20–21, 46–49, 54, 66, 76
Proton-pump inhibitors (PPI). *See* Medications and tests, negative side effects of.
Pseudoephedrine. *See* Medications and tests, negative side effects of.
PTH. *See* Parathyroid hormone.

R

RAA system. *See* Renin-angiotensin-aldosterone system.
Renin-angiotensin-aldosterone (RAA) system, 7–8, 42, 47, 49
Renin inhibitors, 55. *See also* Renin-angiotensin-aldosterone system.

S

Shortness of breath. *See* Anemia.
Sleep
abnormal patterns of. *See* Uremic symptoms.
apnea, 57–58, 91, 97–98
See also Kidney health, improvement of.
Smoking, quitting. *See* Kidney health, improvement of.
Social worker. *See* Case manager.
Sodium. *See* Diet, effects of, on kidney health.
Spirulina supplements. *See* Supplements, effects of.
Spiritual and emotional therapies. *See* Complementary therapies.
Stenosis, 59

Stress reduction. *See* Kidney health, improvement of.

Supplements, effects of
  alpha lipoic acid (ALA), 130–131
  body-building, 101
  calcium, 130–131
  coenzyme Q$_{10}$, 130
  herbal, 136–143
  magnesium, 130
  omega-3 fatty acid, 131
  potassium, 130
  probiotic, 145
  spirulina, 132–133
  vitamin B, 126–127
  vitamin C, 127–128
  vitamin D, 128
  vitamin E, 128–129
  vitamin K2, 129
  weight loss, 101

Swelling. *See* Edema.

Symptoms of kidney disease. *See* Kidney disease.

Symptoms of kidney failure. *See* Uremic symptoms.

T

Tests and medications, negative side effects of. *See* Medications and tests, negative side effects of.

Tests of kidney function
  blood urea nitrogen (BUN), 15
  CAT scan, 16
  creatinine, 14
  electronic GFR (eGFR), 13, 22
  glomerular filtration rate (GFR), 13, 19–20
  Magnetic Resonance Imaging (MRI), 16, 80, 82–83
  ultrasound, 16, 61, 71–73
  urinalysis, 15, 20

TGF-beta. *See* Transforming growth factor-beta.

Toxins. *See* Environmental toxins.

Transforming growth factor (TGF)-beta, 39, 42, 47

Transplant, 23–25

Triglycerides, 50

U

Uremic symptoms, 13

Urinalysis, 15, 20

Urinary incontinence. *See* Incontinence.

Urinary tract
  diagram of, 6
  infection of (UTI), 11–12, 15
  blockage of, 72–73

Urine tests. *See* Urinalysis.

Urologist, 11

UTI. *See* Urinary tract.

V

Vascular disease. *See* Atherosclerosis.

Vasculitis, 65–67
  treatment of, 69

Vitamin B. *See* Supplements, effects of.

Vitamin C. *See* Supplements, effects of.

Vitamin D, 8, 22, 86. *See also* Supplements, effects of.

Vitamin E. *See* Supplements, effects of.

Vitamin K2. *See* Supplements, effects of.

Vomiting. *See* Uremic symptoms.

W

Water, drinking, effect on kidney disease, 102–104

Weakness. *See* Anemia.

Wegener's disease, 67

Weight loss supplements. *See* Supplements, effects of.